Praise for *Whole Body*
The Future of Good Health

In *Whole Body Vibration,* Becky Chambers explains the considerable science behind vibrating for health. Testosterone and growth hormones increase, and cortisol (stress hormone) decreases significantly! WBV helps reverse osteoporosis, increases leg strength, decreases fat in muscles, and improves bone density of spine and legs. It is equal to resistance training in improving leg strength and performance. *And, most of all, it is energizing!*

—C. Norman Shealy, MD, PhD
President, Holos Institutes of Health Neurosurgeon,
Author, and Worldwide Speaker

I am impressed with how thorough yet easy-to-read this book is, presenting complex information about whole body vibration (WBV) in an accessible and easy-to-read style. I intend to recommend this book and WBV therapy to my associates, and suggest to my clients that they read it. I feel sure that then they will have all the information they need, not only about WBV but all of the supporting lifestyle [changes] necessary for the best results as well. I am also impressed by how many issues a WBV practice addresses!

Becky Chambers is right; WBV has powerful effects all throughout your body, including [reducing] inflammation and detoxification. I was overenthusiastic the first day that I used the platform; I did seven minutes, thinking, "Oh, this is no big deal . . ." Boy was I wrong! Twenty-four hours later, every muscle in my body hurt! I remembered Chambers' book, and took charcoal and began to have relief within twenty minutes. I am grateful for the information in this book; it is deeply helpful, especially for stubborn know-it-alls!

—Rain Juvoli, ND, Retired

Whole Body Vibration is a compelling and entertaining look at the myriad and amazing benefits of WBV. I, myself, use my vibration plate every day because, simply put, *it just makes me feel good.*

—**Frankie Boyer, Radio Personality,**
The Frankie Boyer Show

During more than twenty years of hosting *Strategies for Living Radio,* I've been privileged to talk to many innovators, and Becky Chambers is definitely one of them. Chambers' work has been instrumental in changing the way we look at being "healthy" in the twenty-first century. Pioneers such as Becky Chambers are putting healthcare back where it belongs—in our own hands. Pardon the pun, but I get good vibrations from Becky Chambers and *Whole Body Vibration: The Future of Good Health;* I recommend you read it and consider its important message.

—**David McMillian, LPC-S, LMFT,**
Marriage and Family Therapist

Becky Chambers presents state-of-the-art information on the exciting new technology of whole body vibration in her book *Whole Body Vibration: The Future of Good Health,* and I am happy to endorse it. I have been very impressed with whole body vibration since I first learned about it when looking for treatment for a patient with severe osteoporosis who had no ability to exercise. WBV worked beautifully, resulting in a dramatic increase in bone density for my patient in just one year. The more I learn about WBV, the more impressed I am.

WBV can be used in both sickness and health. It can increase muscle strength and improve muscle tone and influence mood by improving neurotransmitter balance. It can have a positive impact on people with

Metabolic Syndrome (increased blood pressure, high blood sugar levels, excess body fat around the waist, and lipid abnormalities). WBV is used by physical therapists, as well as professional athletes, to help heal injuries and improve conditioning. It even seems to have a positive impact on the endocrine system by increasing testosterone levels and decreasing cortisol levels (suggesting that it can reduce the impact of stress on us). I expect we will see much wider use of WBV in the future.

—**John Bordiuk, MD,**
Internist and Medical Director,
Inner Balance Integrative Medicine

I highly recommend whole body vibration for detoxification, lymphatic health, and bone health in my medical and surgical practice. Becky Chambers' book is a great source of information on this innovative health modality that even patients with significant health conditions find easy to incorporate into their routines.

—**Susan E. Kolb, MD, FACS, ABIHM,**
Plastic Surgeon, Author of
The Naked Truth about Breast Implants,
and Host of *Temple of Health Radio Show*

I had the pleasure of interviewing Becky Chambers on the *Nancy Ferrari Show* last year to talk about her book *Whole Body Vibration: The Future of Good Health,* and I was very impressed with her knowledge and expertise on the technology and benefits of using WBV machines. Becky Chambers' passion about living a healthy life is truly what is needed by us all!

—**Nancy Ferrari, CEO,**
Nancy Ferrari Media and Mentoring

More than ever, many of us are interested in living healthy, vibrant lives—especially as we age—and just like Becky Chambers, my life mission has become about feeling good, feeling strong, and incorporating healthy habits and practices into my everyday life. I am so grateful to Becky Chambers for sharing her knowledge about breakthrough body and mind energy therapies. It certainly gives me hope now and for the future.

—**Ann Quasman,**
Chief Fulfillment Officer and
Creator of *Woman Talk Live* and
the *Conscious Conversations Café*

Having delved into the pages of this remarkable book on whole body vibration therapy, I find myself compelled to sing its praises as a medical professional. The comprehensive insights provided here are not just informative but transformative. The author adeptly navigates the scientific landscape, elucidating how this therapy can wield significant benefits such as muscle strengthening, weight loss, heightened bone density, and an invigorated immune system, to name a few. The idea that all this can be achieved in just 10 minutes a day feels almost too good to be true! But I've seen its benefits first-hand, and I don't ever want to be without my whole body vibration therapy!

—**Elizabeth McKay, M.D., FAAD,**
Board Certified Dermatologist,
Board Certified Mohs Surgeon,
McKay Dermatology & MedSpa, PA

Once again Becky Chambers leads the way in sharing an important message . . . whole body vibration heals! In creating this updated trusted resource, her engaging writing style makes this vital information accessible to all. I regularly recommend whole body vibration to my clients and use her books to teach the ease and simplicity of this profound therapeutic. Thank you, Becky Chambers!

—**Linda S Goggin MD IFMCP, ABFM**
Founder, Feel Good Functional Medicine

The vibration plate has revolutionized the way we approach patient care. Its remarkable benefits have had an impact on our patients' overall well-being. By incorporating this innovative technology into our treatment plans, we have witnessed significant improvements in their strength, balance, and flexibility. This remarkable device not only enhances rehabilitation outcomes but also provides a low-impact, efficient way for patients to achieve their fitness goals. Our patients have expressed their gratitude for the vibration plate's ability to accelerate healing, reduce pain, and enhance their overall quality of life.

We are truly grateful for this incredible tool and the books that Becky Chambers has provided with the latest information about the benefits of vibration. Written in simple and clear language, her books help our patients understand the true science of the vibration plate. We are so happy to have a device that provides positive impact on our patients' health and recovery, and Becky Chambers' books for their inspiration and guidance.

—**Denise Bogard, M.D.**
Well Aging Med
—**Nicole J. Davis RN, BSN,**
NJOY Restored, Health and Aesthetics

Also by Becky Chambers

Whole Body Vibration for Calming Inflammation

Whole Body Vibration for Mental Health:
Natural Methods for Finding Peace Amid Chaos

Whole Body Vibration for Seniors

Homeopathy Plus Whole Body Vibration:
Combining Two Energy Medicines Ignites Healing

Whole Body Vibration

The Future of Good Health

Second Edition

Becky Chambers, BS, MEd

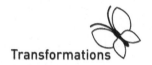

Transformations

Cover design by Darryl Khalil
Model photos by Rick Dorrington, Maddie Freeman
Models: Ula Zielińska, Yuting Qi, Gail Leavitt, Evans Asante
Author photo by Miranda Loud

If you are unable to order this book from your local
bookseller, you may order directly from the author at
her website: www.bcvibranthealth.com.
Library of Congress Control Number: 2023920689

ISBN 979-8-9890679-0-9
Printed on acid-free paper in the United States

To Victor

A challenging gift that led to great growth

Acknowledgments

I want to thank the many people who have helped me learn and write about whole body vibration (WBV). First, I want to thank my many wonderful clients who, over the last twenty-five years, have helped me learn how best to use WBV to help people. I'd like to particularly thank the brave clients who have generously allowed me to use their experiences and names to personalize and enliven this book.

For the photos of WBV in action, I want to thank Ula Zielińska, Gail Leavitt, Evans Asante, Yuting Qi (models), and Rick Dorrington, the photographer.

A heartfelt thanks goes out to my family and friends who have supported and encouraged me throughout the years. Special thanks and love to my mother, Claire V. Smith, who provided editorial skills and financial backing, and to my father who always believed in me no matter how desperate the situation.

I want to thank all the medical professionals who helped me recover and learn about natural health methods, particularly Dr. Keith DeOrio, an early expert in whole body vibration (WBV) and energy medicine. Thank you, Dr. Jaswant Chaddha, for your help and for lending your medical and research expertise to my company's (Vibrant Health) WBV Survey.

I thank Jeanne Mayell for her continuing wise advice in developing this book, including the idea to write the book in the first place!

I thank the following people for their essential and excellent professional services: editor, Sue Vander Hook; interior book designer, Farhan Shahid; cover designer, Darryl Khalil; and publicist, Mary Ann Bohrer.

Author's Note

Like the world itself, the whole body vibration (WBV) field is rapidly changing. Since my last update of this book, there have been many advances in the field of WBV, both in research and on applications, benefits, and technology. That has resulted in better machines.

Our world is sometimes a frightening and challenging place. We must take as good of care of ourselves as possible, physically and mentally, to overcome these challenges, to survive, and to even thrive. Whole body vibration is a critical tool to help you in this quest. It is a powerful way to invigorate your body and mind—strengthening every part of you and boosting your mood and immune system—all in the safety and comfort of your own home.

This Second Edition of *Whole Body Vibration: The Future of Good Health* includes new research on how whole body vibration lowers inflammation and triggers the regeneration of tissues, benefits that apply to most chronic health diseases. New, more versatile machines have also been developed. While once you had to buy two machines to have everything you needed (no matter your state of health or age), now you only need one.

With so much new information—several thousand research studies—and such a broad range of applications, whole body vibration is a topic for more than one book. This book will introduce you to WBV and give you a solid understanding of it and all you need to know to get started with your own whole body vibration program. My other books (see beginning of the book) will provide you with additional information and help with subjects such as using WBV for calming inflammation, for working out, for physical therapy, for seniors and children, for mental health, and as a form of energy medicine.

Contents

Preface

I am a classic "canary in the mine." Fifty years ago, my body began rebelling against the stresses of modern life by developing a host of chronic health issues. Those issues started when I was a young, depressed child and then became chronic and at times severe. They continued for thirty years. I also had crippling insecurities and self-esteem issues. I developed addictive and emotional eating behaviors, including bulimia, and by my early twenties, I weighed 200 pounds. By then, I also had rampant allergies, painful digestive problems, immune system weakness, and numerous disabling joint and nervous system problems.

Back then, I was an isolated freak of nature, but today, what I experienced is becoming commonplace. Chronic health issues are skyrocketing. Nearly fifty years ago I began my search for health and happiness. I hope my hard-earned knowledge and experience saves you time, money, pain, and misery. You may even find joy, love, and success.

I began my search in my teens, using Western medicine and psychiatric care. There was little progress for years, and by my early twenties, the physical complaints urgently demanded attention. Out of desperation, I began considering natural health. Like many people, I grew up believing Western medicine was the only option, so it took me a long time to try other methods. By then, many systems in my body were involved, and the situation was so complex that I was a difficult case.

For example, I had a terrible case of *Candida* (yeast) overgrowth. This is a gut flora disorder that in severe cases can become systemic, causing multiple symptoms and great distress. I would improve with diet changes, products, or drugs to control the yeast. But within weeks, I would be sick again because I had become allergic to whatever product I was taking. Because of this extreme reaction, I was called a "universal reactor" and eventually ended up allergic to more than 300 different foods. For many years, I could only eat by taking daily allergy desensitization drops and rotating all foods so no food was repeated within a five-day period.

I tried many natural health approaches and saw many doctors. My treatment included special diets, nutritional supplements, herbs, Chinese medicine, chiropractic care, acupuncture, homeopathy, heavy metal removal by intravenous and oral chelation, allergy desensitization, and more. But I was still going downhill. By my thirties, I could barely eat anything and had lost 80 pounds, ending up a slim 120 pounds of unhealthy, depressed, and lonely misery.

My immune system was so overworked and weak that the slightest nick in my skin would inevitably lead to an infection that took months to heal. My liver was so overwhelmed that I developed multiple chemical sensitivity (MCS). I could eat only organic food and could not tolerate drugs of any kind. I thought I would eventually get some kind of serious infection and probably die because antibiotics only made me worse.

A key turning point was when I discovered whole body vibration (WBV) about twenty-five years ago and experienced its vast potential to improve health. Using WBV in combination with nutrition, supplements, and homeopathy, I finally began to truly heal. Eventually, I started using WBV in my natural healthcare consulting practice and became the first person in the northeastern part of the United States to use and supply WBV to the public.

Without a doubt, WBV has enormous potential to help people, but like any very powerful instrument, if it isn't used properly, it can cause problems. I have written this book to help people take advantage of the many benefits of WBV without stumbling into the pitfalls. As a natural health practitioner, I have seen that WBV works best when we understand the basic natural health concepts of nutrition, the impact of toxins on our bodies, and chi energy, or our life force.

Introduction

Whole body vibration (WBV) is exploding in popularity worldwide because of its remarkable capacity to enhance health and well-being. WBV has been shown by extensive research over the last fifty years to be intensive exercise. Movement is what we are designed for—it is the true fountain of youth. Still, it is often missing from our busy and sedentary modern lifestyles. As hard as it is to believe without actually experiencing it, ten minutes of WBV training will give you the benefits of one hour of conventional weight lifting, including increased muscle strength, bone density, flexibility, coordination, balance, and weight loss. These benefits alone are enough to drive WBV's popularity, but in fact, they are only the tip of the iceberg when it comes to its total effect on health and well-being.

Ten minutes of WBV training will give you the benefits of one hour of conventional weight lifting, including increased muscle strength, bone density, flexibility, coordination, balance, and weight loss.

WBV machines were initially invented for the Russian space program in the 1970s to counteract the effects of zero gravity and as a training method for their Olympic athletes. In the 1990s, after the Fall of the Iron Curtain, commercial machines were developed and rapidly spread throughout Europe. Ten years later, vibration machines arrived in California and began to be available across the United States. Currently, WBV is predominately known and used for its dramatic effects on the musculoskeletal system, and many companies are making them.

When you stand on a vibration plate, you can feel the vibrations going through your body with a sensation similar to a massage. It seems so simple, but every cell and molecule in your body vibrates, leading to a cascade of effects so astounding that I am regularly met with "It's too good to be true!" It is true and documented extensively by fifty years of research. There are also millions of satisfied users worldwide, including top athletes such as Shaquille O'Neal and Trace Armstrong, sports franchises such as the Denver Broncos and the Miami Dolphins, and celebrities such as Madonna, Clint Eastwood, and Tony Robbins.

Chapter 1 focuses on the effects of vibration on your muscles. All your muscle fibers are activated involuntarily, tightening and relaxing at the same speed the plate is vibrating, twenty to fifty times per second. That effect, plus the increase in gravity as your muscles hold your weight against the vibration, leads to the revolutionary result. Ten minutes of WBV equals one hour of conventional weight lifting.

In Chapter 2, we'll look at one of modern life's most hotly pursued goals—losing weight! Just like traditional exercise, WBV increases your metabolism and muscle strength, which help you burn more calories and lose weight. Cutting-edge research now shows powerful anti-inflammatory effects from WBV, including balancing gut flora with implications for many chronic diseases such as obesity and obesity-related diseases such as diabetes. Just as important, WBV raises serotonin levels, which has powerful antidepressant effects and improves mood and sleep. Since many people overeat for emotional reasons rather than physical hunger, this effect can be critical in the battle to maintain or achieve a healthy weight.

Chapter 3 addresses the issue of bone density loss and WBV's capacity to stimulate bone growth. We know that WBV was originally developed fifty years ago in Russia to counteract the devastating effects of zero gravity on cosmonauts in outer space. And it turns out that vibration transmitted to the bones through muscle is precisely the signal your body needs to increase bone density. This is exciting news for millions in this country and worldwide who are facing the dangers of weakened bones and the lack of safe and effective treatment.

Another life-changing aspect of WBV is described in Chapter 4—its effects on the nervous system and brain. WBV rapidly raises the levels of two neurotransmitters—serotonin and norepinephrine—thus boosting your mood and energy levels. A positive mood strengthens and invigorates your whole body, including your immune system. In addition, exercise has been shown to be the most crucial factor for brain health, powerfully stimulating neural cell growth and strength. This is a godsend for everybody—certainly people facing neurological disease and disability, but truly, *all of us*. Who couldn't use a bit more brain power?

Are you feeling a lack of energy and zest? WBV may be just what you need. Chapter 5 looks at the numerous physiological effects of WBV that increase energy, including rising levels of testosterone (linked to both men's and women's sexual libidos and energy levels). WBV also increases circulation, bringing nutrients and oxygen to all cells. The antidepressant effect also sends new energy through your mind and body.

WBV works in ways similar to acupuncture to stimulate electromagnetic energy. This is acknowledged by Western medicine and

Eastern traditions as being the basis of our neurological system and thus connected to all parts of our bodies.

There's nothing quite like pain to motivate you. If pain is an issue for you, Chapter 6 will be particularly interesting. In this chapter, I focus on the many types of pain that WBV can help alleviate. We'll look at the intriguing question of how WBV can lower pain so quickly and effectively, and how to maximize your results.

Chapter 7 focuses on three common casualties of aging: sex, beauty, and mobility. The rejuvenating effects of WBV on these areas can be attributed in part to increasing levels of stem cells— progenitor cells that can turn into different types of tissues. Another major rejuvenating WBV effect is increasing the human growth hormone, the body's major repair, regrowth, and anti-aging hormone. This effect, plus the increases in testosterone, circulation, and electromagnetic energy, can give you a whole new lease on life.

In Chapter 8, we will look at how WBV stimulates the circulation of your blood and your lymphatic system. Together, these two systems bring nutrients, oxygen, and infection-fighting warrior cells to all your tissues and remove toxins and waste products. WBV has a powerful effect on the lymphatic system, causing so much detoxification that I suggest caution. Start slowly with just a minute or two, and increase gradually. In this case, less is truly more. Can you imagine an exercise program where the biggest problem is doing too much?

In Chapter 9, we will look at the plethora of available WBV machines, the parameters of the various machines, what to look for, and what to avoid. Which one is best for you?

Chapter 10 is a how-to section that gives you specific guidelines (gleaned from my twenty-five years of experience) for achieving the best results with WBV. There is a day-by-day plan for beginners, tips for more challenging workouts for advanced users, and thirty photographs of different exercise, stretching, and massage positions.

WBV is a powerful tool in the search for health and happiness. It has an unprecedented ability to simultaneously work on physical, mental, and energy levels. In a ten-minute session, you can essentially get the benefits of a workout, a massage, acupuncture, and a powerful detoxification treatment, as well as achieve life-changing benefits for many aspects of physical and mental health.

WBV is revolutionary in its capacity to help stimulate your body to heal itself, but also because you are in control. You can do it on your own, in your own home, at your own convenience. There's no need to wait for experts, pay exorbitant sums of money, deal with side effects from prescription drugs, or experience trauma from surgery. I believe there is a place for both Western medicine and natural approaches in healthcare. Consult with your doctor for safety and emergencies, but whenever possible, give your body a chance to heal itself with whole body vibration and other natural methods.

NOTE

The information in this book is not intended to be a substitute for professional medical advice, diagnosis, or treatment. Always seek the advice of your doctor or another qualified health provider if you have a medical condition or have any questions regarding a medical condition or medical symptoms.

Please check the list of whole body vibration contraindications in Appendix 2, and consult your doctor before beginning whole body vibration.

Chapter 1

The Ten-Minute Workout

The Revolution of Whole Body Vibration (WBV)

We all know we should be exercising, right? The problem lies in actually doing it. There was a hilarious ad on TV a while ago about a couple who join a health club but never go. Every day they have a new excuse—too busy, had to work late, too tired, forgot sneakers, lost hairband, mother called! It gets increasingly ridiculous, and we laugh because we've all been there.

But what if exercising was so quick, enjoyable, relaxing, and conveniently located in your own home (or nearby) that it was the highlight of your day? What if you could hardly wait to get to it every day and had to restrain yourself from doing too much? It is possible. Whole body vibration has arrived—and just in time! We are a nation and a world in desperate need of the many life-changing benefits of WBV.

Exercise: The Fountain of Youth

Our bodies are designed for physical activity, and they thrive on it. For example, exercise increases circulation, bringing essential nutrients and oxygen to every body part, including your brain, and removing waste products. Amping up this process helps every cell and organ in your body function at a higher level. And just by exercising, you increase your body's ability to drive the circulatory system. Your heart, which pumps your blood through the arteries on its outgoing journey, becomes stronger. Exercising builds more muscle, which in turn massages the veins in the gentler but essential pumping action that moves the blood on its return trip to the heart. Exercise, whether in a more traditional form or now with WBV, is also critical to maintaining muscle tone, bone density, and a healthy weight.

Our bodies are designed for physical activity, and they thrive on it.

Exercise and Your Brain

Just as important, exercise helps your mood and brain. If you are so depressed and lethargic that you can barely get out of your chair and exercise, your life might seem like an insurmountable mountain. The good news is that the very act of exercising will increase the levels of natural chemicals in your brain called neurotransmitters, which will raise your spirits, energize you, and help your brain function better. Exercise has actually been shown to increase the number of neurons and neural connections in your brain. These are important components of intelligence, so you will actually be getting smarter as you exercise.

TESTIMONIAL

Dear Becky, I could not wait to tell you the great news I received from my doctor. I had my annual blood work done, and my HDL had increased. My doctor was so impressed and happy because the only way to increase it is with exercise. She was praising me and then it dawned on me. I had torn my knee and I was actually doing less exercise. My daughter even got me a walker because I was unable to just walk. Of course, this was not an emergency, and it was during the COVID lockdown, so I had to wait for it to heal. I felt weak from lack of exercise, and my daughter recommended the Vibrant Health Power 1000. I got it, and that was the only exercise I did. I started out slow like you recommended, and it was amazing.

I do standing, sitting, and upper body exercises every day. I felt very calm and centered. It even helped with my depression. My doctor was shocked when I told her I wasn't walking but using my vibration platform instead. She is a big believer in exercising and asked me to send her the website with info on the Power 1000. I cannot wait until my next blood test to see my results. I use it every day to start my day with prayer and meditation. Thanks for such a great product! Woe to the person who interrupts my vibe time!

—Maria A.

The Ten-Minute WBV Workout

Now that you're rearing to go and ready to start your new life as a fit, slim, brilliant citizen of the world, what should you do first? WBV is an excellent place to start, or you can use WBV in addition to any fitness program you already have in place. Why? It is a quick, highly adaptable workout that can be tailored to any level of fitness—from the sedentary couch potato to the occasional jogger, from the tennis player to the weekend warrior, from the amateur athlete all the way to the elite professional competitor.

At the easiest beginner level (and on extra-lazy days), you simply stand on the gently vibrating plate and receive a vibration that will feel like a massage. Through the involuntary automatic activation of your nervous system and thus your muscles, you will be experiencing a mild workout. At the other end of the spectrum, ten minutes of exercising while vibrating equals one hour of conventional weight lifting.

At first that may seem impossible—just too good to be true—but it is true. While the exact ratio does depend on which machine you use and how you use it (whether you work out intensively, gently, or just stand on the plate), forty years of research and the devotion of thousands of

Ten minutes of WBV equals one hour of conventional weight lifting.

professional athletes and elite users, including Shaquille O'Neil, Jane Fonda, Madonna, the Denver Broncos, and the Tennessee Titans, attest to WBV's effectiveness.

TESTIMONIAL

I was mountain biking in the fall of 2017, hit a root, fell off my bike, hit the ground, and fractured my little finger. In the fall of 2018, after using my WBV machine for about four months, I was mountain biking in the same woods and hit a root. This time, as my bike was falling, I was able to jump off and land on my feet. I felt very strong and in control, had increased core strength and balance, and had quad and calf strength. I felt great! I felt like I was an agile twenty-year-old again. Also, a year after using Becky Chambers' Vibrant Health Power 1000 vibration machine, my calves were bigger, evidenced by my ski boot buckles needing to be adjusted! This past ski season in 2019, I had a serious ski fall that could've been deadly; however, no major injuries, no broken bones, and my body healed quickly from bruises and sore muscles and knee! I was fifty-three at the time but felt like a young athlete. Additionally, I want to mention that going through menopause is a great time to use the WBV machine as it helps to maintain muscle tone, which in turn helps boost mood and body image as things begin to shift from changes in hormones.

—Marliana Cataldi, RN, age 53

How Whole Body Vibration Creates Intensive Exercise

♦ Holding weight against vibration increases the effects of gravity. Because of this physical reality (described mathematically as gravity equals mass times acceleration), when suddenly vibrating, your muscles must hold two to three times your actual weight, the exact amount depending on the amplitude of the vibration.

♦ Every muscle fiber will automatically tense and relax at the same rate the machine is vibrating, usually twenty to fifty times per second. That adds up to 1,000 to 3,000 tiny reps per minute—much more work for your muscles than holding a position (static or isometric exercise) or typical repetitive workouts.

♦ One hundred percent of your muscles will be working, while in traditional exercises, only some of your muscles are engaged. For example, in a non-vibrating squat, only about 40 percent of your leg muscles are working. But if you are vibrating, 100 percent of your leg muscles will be firing.

> Holding weight against vibration increases the effects of gravity. Every muscle fiber will automatically tense and relax at the same rate the machine is vibrating, usually twenty to fifty times per second. One hundred percent of your muscle will be working, while in traditional exercises, only some of your muscles are engaged.

The combination of these three factors results in an intensive workout, and by the end of one minute, your muscles may be begging for relief. If it is still not hard enough, you can carry weights, which will rapidly increase the effort as the gravitational force from the vibration doubles or triples the effect of any weight increase.

You can also vary the type of exercise position to change which muscle groups must work to hold your weight. For example, you can do push-ups for upper body strength or sit on the plate in a V shape (see photos in Chapter 10) to work the abdominal muscles. There are endless variations of positions to engage different muscle groups. A typical workout includes one-minute intervals in numerous positions to achieve the effect of a full body workout in ten minutes.

Circulation does increase with WBV, which is partly due to the massaging action of the muscle fibers as they tense and relax. WBV does not provide intensive aerobic exercise, so you should incorporate some type of aerobic exercise in your total fitness plan such as walking, biking, running, swimming, and more. You will probably find it much easier to do that when you are using WBV due to its powerful energizing and mood-elevating effects.

WBV Research for Strength Training

The intense muscle strengthening effect of WBV is clear with younger people,[1] and this effect is a primary reason WBV is used so extensively by athletes around the world. Recent research on using WBV with other populations, especially older people and those with health issues, has been less clear. Some studies are seeing increases in strength, and others are reporting little or no increase.[2]

I believe the problem with this more recent research is that it is not being done properly. The proper type of machine may not be used, and/or there is not a slow enough buildup of time and intensity of the vibration. With the knowledge gained from a lifetime of dealing with health issues, I have had great success using WBV for seniors with health issues. In fact, I find that older, ill, and otherwise less fit and less strong people are the very ones most likely to see dramatic improvements.

In 2019, my company, Vibrant Health, conducted a research survey[3] of our customers using Vibrant Health's Power 1000 machine, which comes with a user manual and my recommendations on how to use it. Ninety percent of the survey respondents were over fifty years of age, and 62 percent were sixty to eighty years old. The survey included fifty-three respondents. The results were unequivocally positive. On average, respondents reported a 25 percent increase in strength and a 28 percent increase in energy within weeks of beginning their WBV program. Almost 20 percent of respondents reported increased strength within a few days of beginning WBV and 49 percent within one month. (See Appendix 1 for a summary of all survey results.)

Respondents reported a 25 percent increase in energy within weeks of beginning their WBV program. Almost 20 percent reported increased strength within a few days, 49 percent within one month.

TESTIMONIAL

I am sixty-eight years young and have had several chronic diagnoses for over thirty years. After over a year of immobility due to low back stenosis pain and chronic hip issues, my biggest concerns were loss of ability, endurance, and vitality. Conventional treatments were not geared for my age and disability from chronic conditions. In the spring of 2018, I started using Becky Chambers' Gentle 500 vibration machine. I felt a boost of confidence in my body and myself as I gained energy and my pain decreased. I consulted with Becky again and upgraded to the Vibrant Health Power 1000 in January 2019. I used to think I was going to end up in a wheelchair; now I am swimming every other day, and I recently added using a light weight lifting machine routine to my gym workouts. The increased confidence from my growing endurance and strength is priceless.

I am forever grateful to have found my way to whole body vibration and Becky Chambers.

—Sandy Gong, age 68

Chapter 2

Losing Weight with Whole Body Vibration

Why Vibration?

Whole body vibration helps you lose weight by speeding up your metabolism, increasing energy levels, elevating your mood, strengthening muscles, lowering inflammation (which is a driving force for many chronic diseases, including obesity), and signaling your body to create bone and muscle rather than fat, even if all you do is stand on the vibrating plate. Scientific research has shown increased weight and fat loss with WBV, along with many other benefits, and my own extensive experience with clients and myself makes it clear that WBV is a huge plus in any weight loss program.

Weight loss is a national obsession, and there are good reasons. It is clear that weight gain and obesity are significant health risks and have a long list of associated diseases. In modern times, with our sedentary lifestyles and easy access to unhealthy but addictive and high-calorie foods, weight gain has become an enormous problem. The psychological toll of this societal obsession can be devastating, and I urge keeping things in perspective. Fat is a natural element of our bodies that is important in small amounts for good health. Historically, fat has been essential to our survival as a species and can make for lovely, soft, smooth contours. However, if you feel you are over your ideal weight and you want to tone your body and lose fat, whole body vibration can help you.

Remember that what is *beautiful* and *attractive* is mostly blooming, vibrant health. That means you'll be around for a long time, creating a wonderful life and helping your loved ones live similarly long, happy lives. The great gift of WBV is that it will help you not only lose weight but also improve your physical and mental health in many other ways at the same time.

How Whole Body Vibration
Helps You Lose Weight

♦ WBV can be an intense workout, and like any workout, it will increase your metabolic rate so you burn more calories and lose weight more easily. And the time required to achieve the same results with traditional exercise is much less. Remember, ten minutes of WBV equals one hour of conventional weight training.

♦ WBV lowers inflammation and balances gut flora,[4,5] which can help you lose weight. Inflammation has been linked to many chronic diseases, including obesity. Gut bacteria have roles in digestion, fat storage, hunger, mood, and food cravings, and all those can significantly impact your weight. Balancing gut flora also calms gut inflammation, which leads to a drop in water retention and bloating, giving you quick improvements on the scale.

♦ Vibration signals progenitor stem cells to develop into bone cells rather than fat cells, leading to leaner muscle mass and bone, and less fat.[6] Stem cells are cells that possess the unique ability to develop into other types of cells, making them an invaluable part of your repair and regeneration systems.

- The workout will also build lean muscle mass by increasing the size and length of your muscle fiber cells. Greater muscle mass will burn more calories all day long. Lean muscle mass can account for 60 percent of your energy and calorie expenditure while at rest.

- WBV raises serotonin levels in your brain, which has a powerful anti-depressant effect (see Chapter 4). With your mental state happier and calmer, it will be easier for you to eat properly and exercise. Everybody knows they should eat well (probably in lesser quantities) and exercise more to lose weight; the problem is actually doing it. WBV helps you be in that calm, relaxed, but energized mental state where you can focus and achieve your goals.

- WBV gives you strength (increased muscle power) and energy (see Chapter 5). So when you do go out to exercise, now more often because you have more energy and are in a better emotional and mental state, you will work harder, consequently burning more calories.

- WBV lowers cortisol levels.[7] Cortisol is a significant stress and aging hormone that promotes fat production and storage. Lowering cortisol levels helps promote fat burning and proper fat metabolism.

- WBV improves joint health and lowers pain in numerous ways (see Chapters 6 and 7) so you have greater mobility and can exercise more.

TESTIMONIALS

I am thrilled with my vibration machine. Combining vibration with diet changes and a Candida yeast program, I have lost forty pounds in six months, after many years of trying to lose weight with little success. My legs are no longer swollen, and I am off my diuretic medication. I also have had high cholesterol my entire adult life (everybody in my family has high cholesterol), and I have been on Lipitor for years. My cholesterol has now dropped eighty points, and I am off Lipitor. My triglycerides were very high (332), and they have dropped over a hundred points to 214. My gas, bloating, and heartburn have disappeared, and my face is clear. The puffiness, poor color, and minor acne are gone.

—Angelica Fiorenza, 57

I've been trying hard to lose weight and tone up for two years, really watching what I eat, working out at the gym and even with a personal trainer for almost a year. I never lost a pound without gaining it right back the next week. Now, after one month, I've lost at least six pounds, and during the holidays too! My clothes all fit much better, and my friends are noticing how toned I am. My daughter poked my stomach last week and said, "Are those your abs? Oh my God!" The biggest thing for me, though, is that I am sleeping! One week after I started, I slept straight through the night, only waking up once. I hadn't done that in ten years, and I am continuing one month later to sleep much better than before.

—Mary Jane Langone

Scientific Research

A 2018 systematic review of eighteen research articles, with a total of 321 human subjects, looked at using WBV with adult overweight and obese patients. The results showed increased metabolism and weight and fat loss, along with improvements in other issues known to be related to obesity such as heart health, peripheral and central circulation, glucose regulation, and inflammation levels. The combined results of these studies led to the conclusion that "six to twelve weeks of WBVT [WBV Training] in obese individuals generally led to a reduction in fat mass and cardiovascular improvements."[8]

Eight studies in the 2018 review reported a body weight decrease from 5–10 percent,[9,10,11,12,13,14,15] with one twenty-four-week study showing continued weight loss. That long-term study, a 2010 study of sixty-one overweight and obese adults, saw significant weight loss with a combination of WBV and diet, with the best long-term

The combined results of these studies led to the conclusioin that "six to twelve weeks of WBVT [WBV Training] in obese individuals generally led to a reduction in fat mass and cardiovascular improvements."

results obtained for those participants who combined WBV with aerobic exercise and diet. Below are their conclusions:

> Combining aerobic exercise or WBV training with caloric restriction can help to achieve a sustained long-term weight loss of 5–10%. These preliminary data show that WBV training may have the potential to reduce VAT [visceral adipose tissue, or fat] more than aerobic exercise in obese adults. . . . Only FITNESS and VIBRATION [participants] managed to maintain a weight loss of 5% or more in the long term.[16]

A 2021 systematic review and meta-analysis of thirteen controlled trials sought to give a definitive answer to the question of whether WBV really works for weight loss. Details of the study can be found in the article "Does Whole Body Vibration Therapy Assist in Reducing Fat Mass or Treating Obesity in Healthy Overweight and Obese Adults?" in the journal *Disability and Rehabilitation.*[17] The conclusion states, "This systematic review and meta-analyses indicate a positive effect of Whole Body Vibration therapy on reducing fat mass (%/kg), especially when combined with conventional weight loss interventions specifically, diet and exercise."[18]

My own research and extensive experience with clients make it clear that WBV is a plus in any weight loss program. In Vibrant Health's 2019 survey using the Vibrant Health Power 1000 machine,[19] 50 percent of those who wanted to lose weight reported that they did, indeed, lose weight. This is a high success rate in an area where success rates are usually low. Our research aligns with other research that show modest but long-term weight loss with WBV.

TESTIMONIAL

I feel like I have always been trying to lose weight. . . . Then, two years ago, my daughter came home from college and said she was going to lose some weight over the summer. I decided to join her. To my utter dismay I weighed in at 178 pounds—way too much for my 5' 2" petite frame. At first, I struggled to lose any weight. After reading Becky Chambers' book, I purchased the Power 1000 vibration machine and began to lose some weight. But then, right before COVID hit, I fell and broke my arm; then came COVID and I lost my job after 24 years with the company. My father died a month later, and I realized this was a lot of traumas all at once. I decided to look at the time off as a blessing and focus on taking care of myself.

I got serious. . . . I went to see a functional medicine doctor who helped balance my hormones, I ate a very clean diet and exercised every day, and I vibrated every day for fifteen minutes and incorporated a dry sauna into my routine. I am happy to report, two years later, that I now weigh 128 pounds – a loss of 50 pounds! My daughter says I am aging backwards!

I really believe the Power 1000 was instrumental in helping me lose wight and keep it off, and a side benefit of vibrating every day is that the pain in my feet and ankles that I was plagued with for years is gone. I noticed that the pain was gone around two months after

> I started using my machine daily. I was out walking with my son, and he asked me how my foot pain was, and I realized it was gone, TOTALLY!
>
> Thank you, Becky Chambers, for your dedication. You have really helped turn my life around. I am so looking forward to your next book!
>
> —Sandy O'Brien, age 58

The early studies with animals and WBV are very encouraging. In one of those studies in 2007, mice that received fifteen minutes of daily vibration for fourteen weeks ended up with 27 percent lower amounts of fat and corresponding increases in bone density than the control mice that didn't get any vibration.[20] In the photos from this study, the dark areas are fat. As you can see, the mice who received vibration are visibly considerably leaner and have fewer dark fat areas.

Mice Exposed to Vibration   Normal Mice

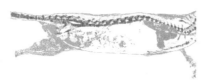   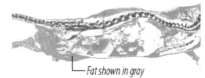

Fat shown in gray

Source: Clinton Rubin; PNAS. Used by permission of Dr. Clinton Rubin. *The New York Times*

This research was done with an extremely gentle type of vibration called low intensity vibration (LIV), which is barely noticeable except in your feet. This is not an intense workout, which led to the discovery that vibration signals stem cells in your bone marrow to turn into bone-building osteoblast cells rather than fat cells.[21] As many of us have experienced, a sedentary lifestyle and a poor diet send these critical stem cells in the opposite, fat-producing direction.

Vibration signals stem cells in your bone marrow to turn into bone-building osteoblast cells rather than fat cells.

This extremely gentle type of vibration does not provide an intense workout, which is more helpful for weight loss. For older or more fragile people who cannot use a more powerful machine, LIV is a good option (see also Chapter 3: Increasing Bone Density).

Inflammation and Hormonal Changes

Recent research on the effects of whole body vibration on gut flora and inflammation levels in the body has triggered a surge of new research since there are implications for many chronic diseases. Chronic inflammation is recognized as a driving force in health conditions as diverse as obesity, diabetes, heart disease, hypertension, arthritis, autoimmune diseases, allergies, asthma, Alzheimer's, numerous digestive issues, and others.[22]

In 2017, there was great excitement when researchers Meghan E. McGee-Lawrence and colleagues at the Medical College of Georgia in Augusta showed that inflammation markers were significantly reduced in type 2 diabetic mice.[23] Those results confirmed similar results in an earlier study.[24] *Science* magazine, one of the most highly respected scientific journals in the country, greeted the new research with a hopeful article that reported, "Now, a new study of obese mice reveals that whole body vibration provides similar metabolic benefits as walking on a treadmill, suggesting it may be useful for treating obesity and type II diabetes."[25]

Whole body vibration improves gut flora in the digestive system and key immune system cells in the gut (M2 macrophages) that produce anti-inflammatory molecules such as the anti-inflammatory cytokine, interleukin-10 (IL-10).[26]

Beneficial changes in the gut are like knocking over the first in a row of dominos since gut health is one of the major origins of inflammation. Gut inflammatory diseases will be alleviated by these changes, but the results also have implications for diabetes and obesity,[27] as well as many other serious diseases driven by inflammation.

A study by the U.S. Military released in 2020 compared the anti-inflammation and regenerative healing effects of WBV to that of standard exercise and found WBV to be superior in several important areas. Inflammation marker levels for IL-10 and IL-6 improved significantly with WBV. Lesser effects were seen with either exercise alone or exercise and WBV.[28]

Whole body vibration improves gut flora in the digestive system and key immune system cells in the gut. The results have implications for diabetes and obesity, as well as many other serious diseases driven by inflammation.

The large 2018 review of obesity research mentioned earlier also reported a large decrease in fasting insulin levels, which indicates improving insulin and glucose metabolism, lowering the risk of insulin resistance, prediabetic and diabetic conditions, high blood sugar levels, and hyperglycemia.[29]

Leptin and adiponectin levels (two other hormones important for weight loss) also became more balanced. Leptin, which decreased, is involved in appetite regulation and thermogenesis (heat production), and it is typically elevated in obese people. Adiponectin, another hormone that helps control glucose regulation and fatty acid oxidation (generally low in obese patients), increased. Improvements in these hormone levels help reduce body weight and fat.

TESTIMONIALS

Becky Chambers combines vast knowledge and experience. In just a couple of weeks with the help of whole body vibration, her counseling, changing my diet, and restoring balance to my gut flora, I actually woke up feeling great, and three inches were off my waist too! Over the next four months, with continuing my program of counseling and WBV, I've lost a total of forty-five previously very stubborn pounds and five inches off my waist, and my mood and energy are better than ever.

—Dr. D. L. Camhi, chiropractor, age 60

I tried everything in the last six months. I was running and doing aerobics. I changed my diet. I even had a personal trainer, and I never lost more than one or two pounds without it coming right back the next week. Since starting at Vibrant Health, in three weeks I lost fourteen pounds, and I feel healthier.

—Andrea Higgins

Troubleshooting

While I have seen excellent results with many clients and myself (once 200 pounds and now 120 for many years), there can be other issues that need to be addressed. If you are not losing weight and inches while using WBV, aerobically exercising, and eating a healthy diet, possible reasons include the following:

1. **Too much vibration too soon:** This is the most common mistake. Vibration is a very powerful detoxification system (see Chapter 8), so many people need to start at just one minute on a gentle machine and slowly build up the time and vibration frequency. Too much vibration too soon can stress your body and lead to temporary detoxification overload so you do not see the beneficial effects. Though it is hard to believe, the first thing to try if you are not seeing weight loss is to vibrate less. Everybody wants to vibrate more, thinking more exercise will help. But in this case, less is more because the detoxification effect is so significant. I see the best results with my clients when we start with one minute and increase slowly.

2. **Candida yeast:** Candida yeast overgrowth is an epidemic in this country and can cause gas, bloating, and water retention, as well as sugar and carbohydrate cravings and many other symptoms (see Resources and Additional Reading for further information). Used properly, WBV will help eliminate yeast because WBV is such a powerful health-enhancing system. **The more you strengthen your overall health, which is linked to your immune system, the less yeast and other bacterial or viral pathogens will be able to survive.** But because WBV is also

> *Everybody wants to vibrate more, thinking more exercise will help. But in this case, because the detoxification effect is so great, less is more.*

a powerful detoxification system that can create stress for your body, too much WBV can temporarily weaken your immune system, leading to yeast levels increasing, along with the associated symptoms.

So again, it is important to start with just a small amount of WBV, sometimes just thirty seconds to one minute a day, and increase slowly. Exactly how much WBV a person will be able to tolerate without aggravating their symptoms varies greatly depending on their overall state of health and the amount of toxicity in their tissues. Thus, it's useful to work with a qualified professional.

3. *Hormonal and metabolic imbalances:* If you have eliminated the first two reasons, which are most likely the causes for not losing weight, you are left with hormonal and metabolic imbalances. Numerous hormonal and metabolic issues can make it difficult to lose weight. (Consult the Resources and Additional Reading list and/or a qualified health professional to address these issues.)

Chapter 3

Increasing Bone Density

Building Bone Safely and Naturally

WBV is famous for promoting bone growth. Over the last forty years, extensive research has shown that WBV safely promotes and increases bone density, more so than conventional exercise that has long been understood to be essential for healthy bone development. This breakthrough is of critical importance to space travelers who lose bone density at a rate up to 100 times faster than a normal person on Earth.[30] It is also important for postmenopausal women in developed countries who are experiencing epidemic levels of bone loss. Add to this scenario the very real dangers associated with bone density drugs, and you have a life-saving technology that has spurred hundreds of studies and interest worldwide.

Research results with animals and younger people have been dramatic. The development and use of vibration in the 1970s allowed Russian cosmonauts to be in space twice as long as their nonvibrating American counterparts (approximately 200 days versus 100 days). More recently, a NASA website cited the effects of vibration on turkeys, sheep, and rats as "profound," and stated that "only 10 minutes per day of vibration therapy promoted near-normal rates of bone formation in rats"[31] under laboratory conditions simulating the zero gravity conditions of space flight. In other research, Dr. Clinton Rubin, Director of the Center for Biotechnology at Stony Brook University, reported decreasing fat in mice by nearly 30 percent and a corresponding increase in bone density with vibration for fifteen minutes a day for fifteen weeks.[32] A research study with a well-trained cyclist showed an increase in bone density of 1.6 percent in just ten weeks.[33]

Since then, there have been numerous studies to pinpoint the best approach for increasing bone density, especially for the populations that need it most such as postmenopausal women and older men, as well as people with health conditions, which led to greater bone loss due to lower activity levels with conditions such as rheumatoid arthritis[34] and cerebral palsy.[35] A large 2018 systematic review and meta-analysis of the subject that focused on ten clinical trials concluded that "WBV is an effective method to improve lumbar spine BMD [bone mineral density] in postmenopausal and older women and to enhance femoral neck BMD in postmenopausal women younger than 65 years."[36]

This study concluded that to achieve the best results, a stronger vibration was best and that the frequency should be at least 20 Hz, the amplitude at least 5 mm, a g-force of 8 gs, and the vibration should be used over a long period (more than 108 sessions).[37]

Searching for these amplitude and g-force numbers when looking for a machine can be counterproductive and confusing, however, since market pressures have led to some companies reporting misleading information (see Chapter 9). Research, like Western medicine, sometimes may also focus intensely on one health issue, disregarding considerations that are important to the whole person. Exactly what type of vibration is best for increasing bone *while still achieving the best overall results* remains uncertain. In Vibrant Health's

2019 survey,[38] 40 percent of respondents (predominantly older and concerned with bone loss) reported either increased or maintained bone density. These results were obtained using the Vibrant Health Power 1000 vibration machine, which has a lower amplitude and g-force than recommended in the reviewed study discussed above.

Vibrant Health's survey results for strength, energy, pain reduction, mobility, mood, and sleep are much better than reported in other research, while the bone-density results appear similar. Thus, for *total health*, including lowering inflammation and pain levels, and brain health, I recommend using a high frequency, mid-range amplitude and g-force, vertical motion vibration machine. Larger, more powerful machines are often too stressful for the body and mind to promote optimal healing (see Chapters 4 and 5).

TESTIMONIAL

I was diagnosed with osteopenia about ten years ago. A white male in my mid-60s, this came as quite a shock. Of course, the docs wanted to put me on a regimen of prescription drugs that warned of side effects worse than softening bones. I decided to go on a regimen of weightlifting instead. I joined a health club, and over the next ten years, I increased my visits to three days weekly, lifting a combined total of over 50K pounds during an hour. I returned to the rheumatologist for another scan in 2019. Hardly any change was noted. But at least I was holding my own instead of getting worse. Then COVID hit, and the gym closed. I began searching for a home alternative. I happened upon vibration therapy about this time and thought I would try it. So I bought a cheap machine for $100 that oscillated. I had only used it for a short time when Becky Chambers published her book *Whole Body Vibrations for Seniors.* What I read there made sense. I decided to scrap the oscillator and invest in the Vibrant Health Power 1000 and bought it from Amazon in June 2020. I followed Becky Chambers' guidance and started slowly increasing my time on the machine to twenty minutes daily after about four months usage. The first improvement I perceived was the loss of the usual aches and pains that I had for years. Next, I realized that despite the absence of strenuous exercising at the gym, I seemed to be maintaining my vigor and stamina. In short, I was feeling great! In 2021, after a year of using the Power 1000 and now at age 74, I went back to the rheumatologist for another scan. She found that I "had clear bone density gains at the three most important sites since 2019 (total spine, total hip and femoral neck)." I told her about the Power 1000. She was familiar with the concept and promised to read up on it. Needless to say, my investment paid off. Best money I ever spent!

—David Anderson, age 74

Protection from Falls

Research with older people and WBV shows improvements in balance along with bone density mass increases. A 2018 study that included the results of seven other systematic reviews about WBV and bone density concluded that WBV enhances muscle strength and balance and helps prevent falls. This large review of studies also found that the results for increasing bone density were not consistent. Later in this chapter, we will talk more about how to best achieve greater bone density, but averting disastrous falls is an excellent outcome in itself. This study summarized the results as follows:

> Training with vibrating platforms is reported to have effect on enhancing muscle strength, improving balance, and reducing the risk of fall in osteoporotic patients, while controversial findings on improvement of BMD in different sites were reported.[39]

TESTIMONIAL

Huge improvement in balance and overall health. Before my purchase of a whole body vibration machine, I read two of Becky Chambers' books so I could be an informed buyer. Per her advice I started out just sitting in a chair with my feet on the vibration machine for thirty seconds. This was due to my age (73) and loss of balance and six falls in six months. As I slowly increased the time, I recently have been able to stand on it for ten minutes per day. That progress took from June to September. In the past two weeks I have been able to walk around without my cane. It is wonderful to regain what I thought was lost. I expect continued improvement as I keep on with my WBV program. Do your research, an do use the machine. You won't be sorry.

—Donna Fought, age 73

Studies with animals and younger people demonstrate clearly that WBV does stimulate bone to increase its density, but building bone is a complex process involving the healthy functioning of many different systems. As people age, many systems in their bodies do not work as well, so just providing the signal to build bone may not be a sufficient intervention.

One critical missing element in the studies with older people is comprehensive nutritional supplementation. Studies on bone density typically provide participants with, at most, calcium, magnesium, and vitamin D. Still, building bone is a complex process requiring more than a dozen critical nutrients. Older people often have decreased nutrient intake and absorption.

One of my clients who received more extensive nutritional supplementation and WBV saw impressive results. Four DEXA bone density scans over five years (all at the same hospital using the same equipment) clearly documented her progress. Mary Onorato was a 70-year-old woman whose doctor told her that going over a bump in the road or coughing too hard could cause a fracture in her vertebrae because her bone density test put her in the category of "extremely severe" bone density loss. Mary experienced a *complete reversal* of bone loss. After two and a half years, she had the bones of a healthy young woman.[40]

Mary Onorato's Lumbar Spine Bone Density

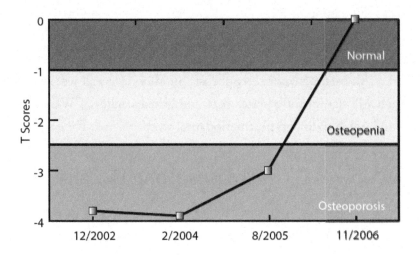

After two years of slowly declining bone density, despite a strict routine of comprehensive mineral and vitamin supplementation and regular weightlifting and walking, Mary found me and began WBV. At that point, she saw a sudden and dramatic turnaround (see graph).

> *NOTE*
>
> *In 2005, Mary switched from a high amplitude double motor vibration machine to the more mid-range amplitude Vibrant Health Power 1000 machine. At that point, her bone density began to increase even more rapidly.*

Mary never took any bone-building prescription drugs and had stopped weight lifting and walking several months prior to beginning WBV, but she always continued her nutritional supplements. The only change in her program was switching from conventional weight lifting to WBV, making it clear that WBV provides a powerful signal to your body to build bone.

Mary's results are not typical, but I wanted to show her results because they are so well documented and clear. Most of my menopausal clients with osteopenia or osteoporosis build bone at a slower rate although still significantly better than published studies of WBV's effect on bone building in postmenopausal women.

How WBV Increases Bone Density

Research by Dr. Clinton T. Rubin through his work with Marodyne Medical and the LivMD low intensity vibration (LIV) device has shown that small, high-frequency signals, a sort of buzz or vibration received from muscle attachments to bone, can cause bone to grow.[41] Previously, it was thought that high-impact signals were needed to trigger bone growth as would be created by the impact of a person's foot against the ground. But it turns out that the quivering of muscle fibers against bone as they contract in the process of running—or from vibration—signals bones to increase in density.

WBV provides small high-frequency signals to many areas and bones intensively, all at once, and with minimal effort. Just standing on a vibrating plate will cause all muscle fibers to involuntarily contract and release twenty to fifty times per second.

WBV provides this same type of small high-frequency signals to many areas and bones intensively, all at once, and with minimal effort. Simply standing on a vibrating plate will cause all muscle fibers connected to weight-bearing bone to involuntarily contract and release twenty to fifty times per second. Different positions are recommended for impacting the arms, hands, wrists, and shoulders (e.g., a push-up) to activate muscles attached to these bones.

The power and size of the vibration machine affect muscle activation and thus the bone density signaling with a greater amplitude vibration, transmitting the signal through more of the body. But very powerful, double motor machines are not necessarily the best choice for your entire body when also considering inflammation levels and your brain (see an explanation of double motor machines below and in Chapters 4 and 9). These machines are also large, heavy, and expensive. Hence, they are not the best choice for many people.

DOUBLE MOTOR VIBRATING MACHINES

To achieve greater power, thus a greater workout effect, many WBV machines have two motors in them. However, it is nearly impossible to completely synchronize two motors. That may result in an asynchronous signal being sent into your nervous system and energy field, which might affect the synchronization of brain waves (see Chapter 4).

On the other hand, extremely gentle vibration such as the low intensity vibration (LIV) (see above) has not been shown to build bone effectively throughout the body for the population who needs it most—postmenopausal women. LIV has been shown to increase bone density in animals—mice,[42] rats,[43] turkeys,[44] and sheep[45]—as well as children with various health conditions.[46,47,48] However, these studies are with young subjects (animals or children), and bone building gets considerably harder with age. These research subjects were also smaller in size than adult people (especially the mice and rats), and gentle vibration will travel through the whole body of small subjects much more easily.

The issue of what magnitude or g-force vibration is best to use for bone density and WBV in general is tricky, and the health and age of the person using the vibration should also be considered. A new 2023 large, systematic review of bone density research that included twenty-three research studies using varying types of vibration concluded the following with a recommendation of LIV vibration for postmenopausal women:

> At this time, considering the high quality of evidence, it is possible to recommend WBV using high frequency (≈ 30 Hz), low magnitude (≈ 0.3 g), and high cumulative dose (≈ 7000 min) to improve lumbar spine aBMD in postmenopausal women. Other parameters [i.e. types of vibration], although promising, need to be better investigated, considering, when applicable, the safety of the participants, especially in vibrations with higher magnitudes (≥ 1 g).[49]

However, this same research also confirmed a greater effectiveness of high frequency, high magnitude vibration for increasing bone density, listing it as the only form of vibration that led to increases in bone density in all three of the bone areas tested: lumbar spine, hip, and femoral neck.

And while LIV has been shown in several studies with adults to "reduce bone loss,"[50,51,52] reducing bone loss means slowing the rate of bone loss, not actually gaining bone density. Actually gaining bone density with postmenopausal women and older men is something that studies with LIV have not yet been able to show.

Thus, for reasons of both effectiveness and safety, I recommend high frequency, *moderate* gravitational force (1.0 g) vibration for most people. If a person cannot handle that much vibration (see Appendix 2 for contraindications that include severe bone loss), starting with very gentle LIV vibration and working your way up is a good recommendation (see Chapter 9 for more on parameters of vibration and choosing a machine).

TESTIMONIAL

My doctor said it was impossible to build bone density at my age and wanted me to take Fosamax. The side effects concerned me. I did research and wanted to try a more natural approach to see if it could make a difference. I decided to do my own experiment and see if a vibration plate would make a difference. I'm excited to report my results. My only change has been using the Vibrant Health Power 1000 Vertical Vibration Platform Machine. For the past six months after purchasing, I used it one to two times a day for five minutes each session. My results are below:

After fracturing two elbows, I had a bone density DXA scan on 9/28/20 showing:

osteoporosis, age 63

Lumbar Spine T-score +0.5

Hip T-score -2.0 osteopenia

Femoral Neck -2.9 osteoporosis

My follow-up scan on 7/30/21 had amazingly improved. Age now: 64 years old:

Lumbar Spine T-score = +0.8,

Normal improvement of 0.3

Hip T-score -1.6, improvement of 0.4

Femoral Neck T-Score - 2.3 osteopenia,
    improvement of 0.6

Went from osteoporosis to osteopenia in six months. Pretty incredible considering the doctor said it wouldn't be possible. Well worth the money for this type of improvement!

I'll stick with the natural method and let them keep the meds and side effects.

—P. Weber, Age 64

Bone Density Drugs

Poor nutrition, a lack of exercise, and the use of numerous drugs that inhibit proper digestion and assimilations of nutrients or bone development have combined to create an epidemic of weak, brittle bones. Statistically, in the United States, one-third of women and one-sixth of men will experience a hip bone fracture at some point in their lifetimes, and these types of fractures often result in death or permanent loss of independence and mobility.[53]

In response, the pharmaceutical industry and Western medicine have developed and heavily promoted a class of drugs called bisphosphonates. They include drugs advertised on television by poorly informed

Fosamax, Actonel, Boniva, and Reclast achieve an increase in bone density by halting your body's natural ability to reabsorb old and damaged bone.

movie stars and celebrities on TV—drugs such as Fosamax, Actonel, Boniva, and Reclast. With use, these drugs do result in bone density tests showing an increase in bone density, but beware! They achieve an increase in bone density by halting your body's natural ability to reabsorb old, damaged bone. The result is more bone, but it is weak, old, and fragile bone.

The situation is most acute in the jawbone where increased blood flow supports the extra bone repair that is normal in that area. This causes a concentration of the drugs and their effects and has led to a surge in cases of a horrifying condition called osteonecrosis (bone death) of the jaw (ONJ). Unfortunately, this process of bone death and rot is usually painless and hidden, so it goes unnoticed for years until the person goes to the dentist for a surgical procedure. Then, with exposure to the bacteria in the mouth and the increased demand for healing, a major disaster follows with permanent, untreatable pain, disfigurement, and great difficulty eating.[54]

Another area where this drug-induced bone weakness shows up is in a bizarre type of severe thigh bone fracture that happens without any unusual stress on the bone. People who have been taking bisphosphonates for five or more years (though occasionally this problem shows up within months) end up in emergency rooms with cross-transverse compound fractures of the femur bone from merely standing up or walking.[55] These are very rare occurrences, but they may be about to become more common as hundreds of thousands of Americans who have been on these drugs for many years reach the critical time period.

These drugs are dangerous, and reducing the length of time a person is on them increases their safety. Some of my clients with severe bone density issues who have been on bone density drugs while using very gentle vibration have seen spectacular results (see testimonial below).

I'm happy to say that there is now an ongoing clinical trial focused on using low intensity vibration that will also look at the effect of taking bone density drugs at the same time.[56] The study is mainly focused on the benefits of combining high-intensity resistance and impact training with LIV. Still, some of the participants in this study are also on bone density drugs. The results will be analyzed and correlated with drug use. Hopefully, this research will show that WBV can increase the effect of bone density drugs and lead to safer, shorter, more effective bone density drug protocols.

TESTIMONIAL

I have been researching whole body vibration (WBV) for years, along with my three brothers, all of whom are also doctors, some of them surgeons. Becky Chambers is the expert; she is very knowledgeable and can guide you on how to use this remarkable system. If you use WBV, go slow, and stick with it. Then you will see the light at the end of the tunnel. Chronic illness, inflammation, pain, depression, and anxiety can improve because vibration releases stress by changing hormone levels such as serotonin, cortisol, and endorphins in your brain that are connected to stress, inflammation, pain, and your emotional state. My brothers are amazed at my progress—now they want their own machines!

I am sixty-four years old and have struggled for years

with a lot of joint pain. I have now been using Becky Chambers' vibration machine and following her advice for the last year. I quickly gained energy and felt stronger, both mentally and physically. Pain and inflammation decreased a lot, and I have been able to stop taking painkillers.

I also have severe osteoporosis and have been on Fosamax for years, but I was only ever able to slow the loss of bone density with Fosamax until I added WBV to my program. In this last year, my bone density has improved a stunning 29 percent in my hip and femoral neck, according to my yearly DEXA scans.

One final note: I initially had a large, complex, and potentially carcinogenic cyst on my kidney. This cyst has now shrunk in the last year to only a small, simple cyst, which is no longer a cancer risk. Of course, before trying WBV, you should check the contraindications with your doctor and follow their advice.

These machines are indeed a beacon of hope. I feel safer now because this machine protects me.

—Luz Peguero, MD, age 64

Normal Bone Growth

Healthy bone formation and growth is a complex process involving numerous systems in the body—bone building and remodeling cells within the bone itself, hormones, liver and kidney function, digestive system health, and the presence of plentiful amounts of more than a dozen minerals and vitamins. WBV stimulates your bones through the quivering muscle fibers and also the rest of your body, helping to keep all these systems working at a high level.

Within our bones, one type of specialized bone cell called an osteoclast breaks down old, worn-out bone. Another type of bone cells, osteoblasts, are bone-forming cells that pull calcium, magnesium, and phosphorus from the blood to build new bone. Without osteoclasts, damaged bone builds up, leading to weak bone. Without healthy osteoblast activity, new bone will not form.

Bisphosphonate drugs increase total bone density by killing osteoclast cells. The result is weak and diseased bone. In contrast, WBV signals stem cells in your bone marrow to turn into bone-building osteoblasts rather than fat cells, leading to increased bone density[57] without interfering with removing old, weak bone.

Excellent nutrition and a healthy digestive system that can extract and absorb all the necessary nutrients are critical to building bone. In addition to calcium, magnesium, and phosphorus, it is also necessary to have available the minerals strontium, boron, zinc, manganese, copper, silicon, molybdenum, and selenium, as well as vitamins A, C, D, K1, K2, B6, B12, folate, and riboflavin.[58]

Fortunately, a healthy diet for building bone is the same diet that is healthy for every other part of you. A primarily plant-based, whole-foods diet with small amounts of animal products (if desired) will make an enormous difference in your health. All parts and systems in your body will work better, and the nutrients that every part of your body requires to function will be supplied. In deep and scary contrast is the average American diet with its heavy load of junk food, fast food, and mind-bogglingly tiny amounts of fruits and vegetables.

The second National Health and Nutrition Examination Survey found that only 27 percent of Americans eat three servings of fruits and vegetables per day, including potatoes. Most potatoes were eaten as French fries and potato chips,[59] and they don't count.

An excellent book in which the processes of nutrition, drugs, and bone building are extensively researched and clearly detailed is *Your Bones: How You Can Prevent Osteoporosis & Have Strong Bones for Life Naturally,* by Lara Pizzorno who has written numerous natural health books and publications.

The Role of Stress

Chronic stress is another factor in bone loss that WBV can help. Chronic psychological stress leads to a decrease in bone mass and density through changes in the hormonal and immune systems, which impact the natural bone-building system. Healthy eating and exercise suffer under stress, and activities such as smoking and drinking likely increase stress.[60]

WBV is an effective anti-depressant tool that has been shown to lower stress and improve mood (see Chapter 4), thus addressing a multitude of behaviors and causes of bone loss.

TESTIMONIAL

I am seventy-five years old and taking care of my husband in the final stage of Parkinson's, so taking care of myself is most important for both of us. I have been using WBV for three years, and I do not want to be without it for energy, strengthening muscles, even while doing facial exercises and just feeling good. Another benefit is being thin, 5'4" at 107 pounds and having the beginning of osteoporosis, my bone density has improved from a T-score of -0.75 to -0.65.

I usually do not write reviews, but I really am thankful for this machine. It's convenient and simple to use, and it works.

—Janet G. Harris, age 75

Older People and Bone Growth

As people age, critical systems for bone building may not function as well. Digestion and assimilation of nutrients may be poor, hormonal changes decrease bone building (especially in women), and older people often take drugs that interfere in some way with the process of building bone. For example, people with low stomach acid do not digest and absorb many nutrients (including only about 4 percent of calcium carbonate, the most commonly used form of calcium supplement). Studies have shown that about 40 percent of postmenopausal women are severely deficient in stomach acid.[61]

Even worse, many of these people will end up further compounding the problem by taking antacids (over-the-counter or prescription) for acid reflux when, in fact, the problem is poor digestion due to too little acid, not enough enzymes, or *Candida* yeast overgrowth, all of which could be resolved easily and quickly with natural treatments.[62]

Western medicine is notoriously poor in its understanding and approach to nutrition. While occasionally WBV bone density studies provide calcium and magnesium to participants along with WBV, usually no nutrients are provided. But you cannot build a house with only lumber and nails. You also need nail guns, workers, screws, measuring tools, siding, sheetrock, windows, doors, and more. It is the same with building bone. There are many critical elements, and nothing can happen without them. The vibration supplies the signal, something like a foreman yelling, "Let's go." The calcium and magnesium could be the lumber, but where are the workers, nails, nail guns, and such? You end up with a lot of lumber lying on the ground and a foreman yelling, "Let's go! Let's go!"

Nutritional Supplements

Healthy, whole food choices are important. But even with excellent food choices, our food supply is so compromised by poor soil, overuse of nitrogen fertilizers, early picking, and long shipping and storage times (not to mention food processing that destroys the remaining nutrients) that it can be very difficult to get enough nutrition to reverse existing health issues.

For that reason, I generally recommend taking high-quality nutritional supplements along with eating a healthy diet. An excellent comprehensive mineral and vitamin bone-building supplement that provides more than two dozen nutrients essential for bone growth is a product called ProBono made by Ortho Molecular Products. Another product I recommend (which is considerably less expensive) is a plant-based supplement called Bone Renewal made by Pure Synergy.

Caution: Vitamin D is an essential vitamin for numerous functions in your body, including building strong bones, strengthening your immune system, and maintaining a stable mood. But Vitamin D is also toxic at high levels and can cause kidney damage and bone loss instead of stronger bones. It is easy to take too much Vitamin D by mistake since it has gotten very popular over the last ten to twenty years and is now included in many supplements. Check for Vitamin D in all your supplements. If you have been taking more than the National Institute of Health's (NIH's) recommended amount of 600–800 IUs per day (for an adult),[63] especially over a period of years, check with your doctor who can test for toxic levels of Vitamin D in your blood.

Chapter 4

Get Smart, and Protect Your Brain

A Wondrous Gift

Your brain, home of your mind and soul, connects you to the universe and makes you a unique being of vast potential and ability. Through your mind and soul, you link to the knowledge of people everywhere throughout time—every aspect of the world around you, your own body, and your existence. Through the nervous system and chi energy, the brain links to every organ, system, and molecule in the body. Thus, key to reaching your potential and building a rewarding life is to stimulate your brain and keep it healthy and vibrant well into old age.

The latest research is that nothing helps your brain develop and stay healthy more than exercise. The article "Jogging Your Brain" in *The New York Times Magazine* states, "For more than a decade, neuroscientists and physiologists have been gathering evidence of the beneficial relationship between exercise and brainpower. But the newest findings make it clear that this isn't just a relationship; it is the relationship. . . . Exercise, the latest neuroscience suggests, does more to bolster thinking than thinking does."[64]

WBV has been proven beyond a doubt to be intensive exercise when used for that purpose. Hundreds of research studies, top athletes around the world, and, in fact, anybody who has ever tried working out on a powerful vibration plate with mus-

> *"Exercise, the latest neuroscience suggests, does more to bolster thinking than thinking does."*

cles begging for relief can attest to this. Even if you only stand on a vibrating plate, you will be stimulating muscles to contract and neurons to fire twenty to fifty times per second, which adds up to 10–15 thousand times in one ten-minute session—massive neurological stimulation.

With a wide variety of possible positions on the plate and intensities of vibration, WBV can be adapted for all levels of physical ability. That allows almost anybody, from a pro athlete to a wheelchair-bound person, from a busy professional to a depressed and unmotivated low achiever, to experience the neurological and other benefits of exercise.

A Complex, Intricate Organ

Your brain contains 100–200 billion neurons (nerve cells). Each neuron connects to as many as 1,000 other neurons through dendrites (thin nerve tissue filaments) that make up a branching tree-like structure. These connections between neurons are called synapses, and there are some 300 trillion synapses in a brain, creating vast networks of interconnected neurons. At each synapse, signals leap across a tiny synaptic gap via natural chemicals called neurotransmitters, activating an electrical signal that shoots through the next neuron. The latest research shows that there are 1,000 activation sites for these neurotransmitters per synapse.

The result is a brain in which there are more neurons than people on Earth, more synapses than stars in our galaxy, and more complexity than all the computers on Earth put together. Stretch out all those dendrites plus axons (the part of the neuron that is something like the trunk of a tree with a root system that connects to organs and tissues up to three feet away), and they would reach to the moon and back.

It is this very complexity, especially the number of connections between neurons, that gives us our intelligence. Thinking involves neurons sending electrochemical signals across the synaptic gaps, thus lighting up pathways throughout that vast network of billions of neurons in your brain.

Whole Body Vibration Is a Powerful Natural Antidepressant

Two neurotransmitters—serotonin and norepinephrine—have been shown to increase with whole body vibration.[65] Serotonin is a critical neurotransmitter in your brain that contributes to sounder sleep and feelings of mastery, pleasure, and relaxation. This is the same neurotransmitter that is targeted by prescription antidepressant drugs such as Prozac and Wellbutrin, as well as many illegal drugs such as marijuana, cocaine, and ecstasy. While prescription drugs for depression can be valuable to help alleviate symptoms, they also have side effects and can lead to increasing tolerance and dependence on those drugs. WBV is a natural, safe, rapid, non-addictive, and legal way to increase serotonin and norepinephrine.

Exercise has long been known to be a powerful way to elevate mood and calm anxiety, and WBV is quick and easy exercise. But not all exercise is the same when it comes to elevating your mood, as a 2021 survey of 17,000 people in China found.[66] This study compared the effect of different types of exercise on mental health during the extreme stress of the COVID lockdowns. Participants were grouped by their level of intensity as well as degree of social interaction. WBV was in the group of moderate intensity exercise systems, which was found to be the most effective for improving mental health. Not surprisingly, exercise that involved social interaction such as family games, group yoga, qi gong, or other exercise systems was also found to be particularly helpful for mental health.

"Exercise, the latest neuroscience suggests, does more to bolster thinking than thinking does."

There is a wealth of evidence linking your emotional state and your immune system. Being depressed or anxious is linked to catching more infections and experiencing the symptoms more strongly. On the other hand, social contact and laughter have been shown to reduce stress hormones, which are linked to your immune system. To improve your WBV results even more, share your WBV discovery, and invite your friends over for a WBV party. Or even better, set up a regular time to work out together, via Zoom if necessary.

"A 2021 survey of 17,000 people in China found that . . . WBV was among the most effective [types of exercise] for improving mental health."

Your emotions have a direct effect on stress hormones such as adrenaline and cortisol, which have wide-ranging effects on the nervous and immune systems, increasing inflammation and stress hormone levels such as cortisol. When stress is prolonged, the effects can be damaging, leading to profound changes in the immune system and making you more susceptible to viruses, bacteria, and other infections. Increased inflammation and stress hormones impact many systems in your body that affect weight loss, bone building, and most chronic diseases. WBV has now been shown to lower the level of inflammation (see Chapters 2 and 3) and cortisol,[67] your major stress hormone.

In today's world where stress and infections are pervasive threats, we must find a way to stay calm and peaceful in the midst of turmoil and fear. This is challenging, but having a WBV machine in your own home can raise your spirits, reduce stress, and improve your immune system—a personal "laughter is the best medicine" device.

Norepinephrine is both a neurotransmitter and a hormone, and low levels of this essential molecule have been linked to depression and low energy. Norepinephrine, along with epinephrine (also known as adrenalin), underlies the fight-or-flight response, giving the body sudden energy in times of stress. It

WBV can raise your spirits, reduce stress, and improve your immune system—a personal "laughter is the best medicine" device.

increases the heart rate, triggers the release of glucose from energy stores, increases blood flow to skeletal muscles and oxygen supply to the brain, and can suppress nerve inflammation. While short-term stress can stimulate the immune system, prolonged stress can have profound negative effects on the immune system. It is essential to have a way to calm down and destress.

Early studies with rats showed rapid increases in serotonin levels with WBV.[68] Subsequent studies with populations such as college students[69] and children,[70] as well as the large Chinese survey mentioned earlier, have confirmed that WBV relieves depression and anxiety. Anecdotal evidence of improved mood with WBV is also strong. Hundreds of my clients and thousands of users around the world report rapid and dramatic improvements in mood, energy, and sleep within days of beginning vibration. They also report increased motivation, focus, and activity levels. This is an area of great potential and should be investigated more thoroughly.

> *Hundreds of my clients report rapid and dramatic improvements in mood, energy, and sleep.*

How Whole Body Vibration Helped My Brain

I spent forty years telling people I couldn't write, that I had terrible writer's block, and was too depressed and repressed to write. This was true for forty years. Writing was a nightmare for most of my life, to the extent that I dropped out of a high school course because I had to write a term paper and couldn't. I majored in biology at college because I liked the subject but also because you didn't have to write papers.

I exercised and used other natural health approaches for years before finding WBV, sometimes exercising extensively (as my health would allow), but those approaches did not noticeably affect my writing issue. Then I began using WBV, and from the time I started vibrating with the *proper type* of vibration about fifteen years ago, my ability to write changed dramatically.

Beginning *the day I started using the proper type of vibration machine,* my writing suddenly began to improve so markedly that I have since written five books, including this one, which has been the best-selling book about WBV in the country since the first edition was released in 2013. Of course, there are other important factors for success as an author, but the dramatic change I saw that day and in the years since has made a believer out of me.

TESTIMONIALS

I really enjoy the vibration – something about it just raises my spirits, and I come off feeling recharged and optimistic, even just doing a standing meditation. I am grateful to have found Becky Chambers, read her book, and followed her advice on how best to begin, because I have not injured myself as has happened in the gym and with PT for me in the past. And I can happily report seeing marked improvements to general health, sleep, stamina, and mood.

—Stephanie Wolford, age 50s

In a nutshell, I am excited to wake up every morning! Sleep is a joy. There is bounce in my step, and I can wear a smile out. Nothing qualifies as a chore, and I have found something in each thing to make it interesting. (Fortunately, my husband does the laundry, so I haven't had to be tested on that score.) It has been a pleasure to live without the stress, weight, and shifting profile I had been coping with. You have put my mind on vacation.

—Doreen Fullmer, 68 years young

Since I started vibrating two months ago, I am so much calmer and happier than I was and sleeping more soundly. My kids say, "Mom, you're definitely less up-tight and angry."

—Monica Calzolari, Director of Enrollment Communi-
cations, University of Massachusetts Boston`

I have become addicted to my vibration plate, even if it's only for a few minutes a day. It's my feel good therapy. A day without vibrating is like a day without sunshine! It just makes you feel so good.

—Frankie Boyer, radio personality

I am happier and have more energy now than I ever did when I was on Prozac.

—Anonymous

I'm like the Energizer Bunny, my hay fever is gone, my mood is better and more stable, I lost thirty pounds, and I am much stronger than I have ever been.

—Doreen Hadge, housecleaner

Neurogenesis and Plasticity

Neurogenesis is the creation of new brain cells. This was once thought to happen only before birth, but it is now known that at a slower pace, neurogenesis does continue throughout life. Neurogenesis allows for brain plasticity, which means your brain can continue to grow and change throughout life, making new neural connections that allow you to not only learn new skills and knowledge but also to increase your ability to learn, produce, and change.

An amazing example of neurogenesis and brain plasticity later in life is a new therapy that has been developed for stroke victims who are paralyzed. Intensive physical therapy for many hours per day with an arm and hand that have been paralyzed for as long as seventeen years—while the normal arm and hand are immobilized—results in the regeneration of brain matter and physical function of the arm and hand.

Exercise triggers neurogenesis by prompting the production of brain-derived neurotropic factor (BDNF), which strengthens cells and axons and the connections among neurons, as well as sparking the formation of new neurons. BDNF is thus the physical mediator, increasing the complexity and strength of the neural network in the brain that reflects intellectual potential.

Research that shows this connection between exercise and the brain has primarily been done with aerobic exercise. However similar neurological and muscular processes are involved with weight lifting type exercises, to which WBV is most similar. Perhaps WBV, with its massive neurological stimulation, will eventually be found to stimulate BDNF and brain development even more effectively than other forms of exercise. We eagerly await scientific research in this area.

Neurological Diseases

There has been a lot of interest—with encouraging results—in using WBV for neurological diseases. Research over a wide range of neurological issues has shown promising results. Research on using WBV has been heating up for everything from movement disorders such as Parkinson's and multiple sclerosis to cognitive issues such as dementia and attention-deficit hyperactivity disorder (ADHD),

A 2019 systematic review of twenty research studies using WBV with a total of 687 people with either stroke, multiple sclerosis, Parkinson's disease, or cerebral palsy concluded that there is a "positive effect of the long-term effect of whole body vibration training on mobility in patients with neurological disorders."[71]

Good outcomes have been seen over a range of different measures for mobility and movement with these conditions. Long-term mobility improved for people with stroke,[72,73] multiple sclerosis,[74] and cerebral palsy.[75] Improvements were seen for Parkinson's disease in balance and postural control, as well as movement tests such as the TUG (Timed Up and Go) test and the 8-Meter Walk test.[76,77] Other studies have reported a positive effect on balance and postural control in patients affected by stroke[78,79,80] and multiple sclerosis.[81]

Other conditions that affect cognitive functions, including ADHD and dementia, are also showing improvements with WBV. A 2014 study with eighty-three healthy individuals and seventeen adults who were diagnosed with ADHD[82] found that "WBV was demonstrated to improve cognitive performance of healthy individuals as well as of individuals with ADHD." Another study with older women with dementia where brain function was monitored with an electroencephalogram (EEG) test and physical movement measures found that "whole body vibration exercise intervention can be a safe and effective exercise method that can increase EEG activation in women with senile dementia and delay and prevent functional decline in their brain."[83]

However, some of the results of the research studies have been conflicting and confusing. A new, large systematic review published in 2022 concluded that "WBV and FMV [focal muscle vibration] appear to play a considerable role in reducing spasticity and improving gait, balance, and motor function in stroke patients" and that "vibration therapy seems to be unable to reduce spasticity in multiple sclerosis and cerebral palsy."[84] Yet the earlier 2019 review included two studies that did report improvements in spasticity for cerebral palsy.[85,86] Other research conflicts as well, such as two studies that failed to find improved mobility as measured by the TUG test and the 6MWT (6 meter walk test) for multiple sclerosis patients.[87,88]

Long-term mobility improved for people with stroke, multiple sclerosis, and cerebral palsy. Improvements were seen for Parkinson's disease in balance and postural control, and movement.

"WBV and FMV [focal muscle vibration] appear to play a considerable role in reducing spasticity and improving gait, balance, and motor function in stroke patients."

Based on my experience, I hypothesize that the conflicting results of the impact of WBV on neurological conditions may be related to the widely varying vibration protocols that are used. There are many variations in the kinds of vibration machines and motions, amplitudes, frequency, and length of time per session.

I recommend high frequency, low amplitude, single motor, vertical vibration, with the goal of delivering a strong, synchronized (see below) yet gentle vibrational message to the neurological system. From my experience dealing with many people with neurological issues over the last twenty-five years, this type of vibration is the most successful.

There is a wide variation in the study protocols, but one major problem is that in general the studies gave elderly people with disease more and sometimes much more vibration than I as an experienced natural health practitioner using WBV would give to that population. For example, one study with disappointing results gave two vibration sessions per day using an oscillation vibration machine (that delivers low frequency, high amplitude vibration) for fifteen minutes per session over a period of three days to elderly people with Parkinson's (average age of seventy-four years). That is a total of seventy-five minutes of vibration in three days.[89]

The benefits of using the best vibration for the brain as well as the body can be seen especially with more fragile people such as those with neurological diseases, but really, don't we all want and need the best vibration for our brain?

I would start elderly people with Parkinson's with low intensity vibration (LIV) (extremely low amplitude, high frequency vibration) for five minutes a day, and gradually increase the speed and time. With so many different variables, it is hard to quantify exactly the difference in magnitude between these two protocols, but it is probably at least a fifty-fold difference. Even in younger people without such severe health issues, I generally see the best results starting with a small amount of time with the right machine and building up slowly over a period of weeks or months, depending on the individual.

I believe that in general, researchers are using too much vibration too soon, and they are using desynchronizing or otherwise stressful-for-the-mind vibration machines to achieve the best results.

Different types of neurological diseases may also need different approaches. My multiple sclerosis people report better results by focusing on working out with the vibration, while the Parkinson's and Alzheimer's people respond to just standing on the plate and the neurological stimulation that provides.

The benefits of using the best vibration for the brain as well as the body can be seen especially with more fragile people such as those with neurological diseases, but really, don't we all want and need the best vibration for our brain?

TESTIMONIALS

I'm dealing with Parkinson's. I was walking like Frankenstein – really stiff! And now, with using my machine, my walking is like butter – I can walk gracefully!

My son noticed; we went on a trip and he said, "You are walking better!" And my neighbor came out, and she said, "You're walking better!" My daughter noticed too.

Recently, I went to the doctor's for the first time in five months, and they said I had lost eight pounds. I said, "That's the machine, it's the machine!"

—Gigi Gregory, age 81

I am thrilled with my vibration machine. I've had multiple sclerosis for nine years and had to give up doing the things I loved because of my difficulties with movement and stability. I quickly saw increases in my strength, coordination, and balance, also my mood and energy level. I feel like I can handle my life and work again. I even ride my bike again and hike in the hills behind my home again. Thank you!

—Mark P, age 57

I have been teaching Pilates for over twenty years. A few years ago, I started researching whole body vibration. I soon found that Becky Chambers is the leading pioneer in this area, and I quickly bought her books and began to recommend and incorporate WBV in my work. For myself, I have adult ADD. When I need to focus and calm my mind, I use WBV with deep breathing, and I find it very valuable.

My brother, age sixty-six, was diagnosed with Parkinson's four years ago. I sent him a WBV plate, but he was a hard sell. He is thrilled! He says his balance and strength are so much better from adding WBV to his workouts! And I feel like I have truly helped him. WBV is a tool I don't hesitate to suggest to my clients!

——Shirley C., age 67

The Future – Super High Frequency Vibrations?

An innovative new approach to vibration and Parkinson's is being pioneered at Stanford University by Peter Tass.[90] Currently, last-ditch Parkinson's treatment has been surgically implanted deep brain electrical stimulation. Dr. Tass's idea was to replace this invasive brain surgery with a very high frequency vibration approach using gloves with vibration only on the fingertips.[91] The idea of delivering a "vibrotactile coordinated reset" is to send a message deep into the brain to "reset" pathological neurological functioning.

This research amplifies to an extreme degree the method I use and recommend—high frequency, low amplitude vibration. The vibrating pads on the fingertips deliver super high frequency vibration (100–300 Hz) at extremely low amplitudes, to people with Parkinson's, and they are getting stunning results. After one treatment, a man who could barely make it from a doorway to a chair is walking freely. Four months later, he is running marathons. Watch before and after video at https://www.today.com/video/new-vibrating-glove-eliminates-parkinson-s-tremor-157390405854 (or google "New vibrating glove eliminates Parkinson's tremor (today.com)).

Research on vibration gloves for Parkinson's is currently in clinical trials, with the hope of a commercial product available in 2024. If you are currently suffering from Parkinson's disease, my suggestion is to start now with the right type of vibration plate (see the Ultimate Vibe in Chapter 10) and add the gloves when they are available. My clients are getting results now for their neurological symptoms.

There are many additional benefits that the stronger vibrations of a vibrating plate bring, including muscle and bone strengthening. The gloves may end up a miracle for some diseases for resetting brain circuitry, but you should still use a whole body vibration. At this point, also keep in mind that only results with Parkinson's disease are being reported at this stage. It is unknown yet how this approach might affect other neurological diseases.

Other research has focused on Alzheimer's disease using sound and light to deliver super high frequency, low amplitude vibrations to the brain.[92] Using a mouse model, researchers at MIT have produced brain scan images showing that Alzheimer's type "plaques were cleared in large swaths of the brain, including areas critical for cognitive functions such as learning and memory."[93]

We may be on the edge of a new era of medicine where healing with the aid of vibration is possible to a degree previously unheard of and without the harm of drug side effects and invasive surgeries.

Brain Synchronization – A Missing Link?

Brain synchronization is the simultaneous, in-phase firing of brain cells across regions of the brain. These combined signals generate electromagnetic brain waves that can be measured by electroencephalography (EEG) and magnetic resonance imaging (MRI).

How does this relate to WBV? Synchronized wavelengths from an outside source can cause "brain entrainment"—the synchronization of brain waves. Brain entrainment has been studied with sound and light and has been linked to increases in creativity, memory, learning, problem solving, and intuition, as well as improvements in depression, anxiety, and ADHD.[i] Biofeedback, for example, takes advantage of brain entrainment to treat mental and physical health issues. There are now numerous companies promoting sound entrainment recordings for better brain function.

---

i   There have been many studies to back these claims. Please see the "Brain Synchronization" section under Additional Research Studies at the back of the book.

In fact, research with WBV with healthy adults and those with ADHD has shown improvements in cognitive function,[94] and there has been exciting results with other brainwave entrainment methods and improvements in Alzheimer's disease.[95]

> Certain types of whole body vibration deliver synchronized signals to the nervous system that I believe may similarly lead to brain entrainment. Single motor vibration machines can produce a smooth, synchronized vibration. However, double (or dual) motor vibration machines can send an asynchronous signal into the nervous system, which will then transmit to your brain. The extent to which these double motor machines could have long-term consequences on your health has yet to be studied. However, I noticed negative impacts on my own health when I used double motor machines. (See my story in the next section.) While synchronized brain waves have been linked to beneficial effects, the opposite state, asynchronous brain-wave activity, has been linked to disease states such as ADD, schizophrenia, depression, traumatic brain injury, and others. As the brain controls the body, theoretically brain desynchronization could affect the physical body as well as mental states.

Synchronized brain waves seem to foster the formation of new synaptic connections, or brain plasticity, and learning. Earl K. Miller, Picower Professor of Neuroscience at MIT and senior author of a study published in *Neuron* in June 2014, has been studying the effects of brain synchronization. According to Dr. Miller in an interview with the MIT news office, he has found that "the phenomenon of brain-wave synchronization likely precedes the changes in synapses, or connections between neurons, believed to underlie learning and long-term memory formation."[96]

Brain plasticity (the formation of new connections between brain cells) has been known for some time to be a critical element for learning. However, brain plasticity—the actual growth of neurons—takes too long to account for the human mind's flexibility. How the brain can process and utilize new information almost instantly has remained a mystery. As Miller explains, "The human mind can rapidly absorb and analyze new information as it flits from thought to thought. These quickly changing brain states may be encoded by synchronization of brain waves across different brain regions. . . . Plasticity doesn't happen on that kind of time scale."[97]

Miller further describes the link between brain-wave resonance and brain development with an intriguing allusion to separate voices joining together; that is, waves of sounds. "There is some unknown mechanism that allows these resonance patterns to form, and these circuits start humming together. That humming may then foster subsequent long-term plasticity changes in the brain, so real anatomical circuits can form. But the first thing that happens is they start humming together."[98]

Brain synchronization also increases with meditation. Dr. Joe Dispenza, an internationally known lecturer, researcher, and author, has been studying and mapping the brain waves of meditators for decades. He describes the effects of brain synchronization, or coherence, like this: "What syncs in the brain begins to link in the brain. Once your brain gets coherent, you get coherent. When it gets orderly, you get orderly; when it works well, you work well."[99]

Dr. Dispenza describes the opposite state—asynchronous brain-wave activity—as one that "causes our brain waves to fire in a very disordered, incoherent pattern (which in turn means our bodies can't work efficiently). . . . the electrochemical messages or signals they are sending to different parts of the brain and body are mixed and erratic, so the body cannot then operate in a balanced, optimal state."[100]

My Experience with Brain Desynchronization

To achieve greater power, thus a greater workout effect, many WBV machines have two motors in them. However, as engineers can attest, it is nearly impossible to synchronize two motors. Thus, double motor machines are likely sending asynchronous signals throughout your body. While people may not consciously detect the millisecond lack of synchronization level when they are on a WBV machine, the nervous system and the body's energy fields are extremely sensitive and are likely able to pick up the lack of synchronization.

My own experience when I first began using WBV twenty-five years ago as the sensitive canary in the mine, was that asynchronous machines led to illness. After my first few months with one of these double motor machines, during which I did see improvements and became stronger than I had been in many years, my health suddenly deteriorated. I experienced a mysterious downturn with severe muscle weakness. My allergies, chemical sensitivities, multiple infections, digestive distress, and nervous-system problems also all returned. It seemed to be linked to the vibration since I would get much worse after the slightest amount of vibration with the double motor machine I was using. This response occurred numerous times as I attempted to resume using WBV. But what exactly about the vibration was bothering me was difficult to determine.

Dr. Keith DeOrio, an early expert in WBV[101] and my doctor at that time, theorized that my sudden downturn was due to a desynchronization effect from the double motor machine I was using at that time. Concerned about my health and unsure if Dr. DeOrio's theory was correct, I chose not to use any WBV for several years. A few years later, I switched to a single motor machine and began to notice health improvements. I have now been exclusively using single motor vertical vibration machines for fifteen years, with my health continually improving.

I believe asynchronous machines (double motor) may be part of the reason some research on WBV with older people and those with health issues has not been as good as expected based on early research with animals and healthy young athletes. Since I use only single motor machines with my clients, it may explain in part why I have had success working with elderly and fragile people. My machines do not send asynchronous signals to the body and brain.

My hypothesis that using a fully synchronized vibration can improve the results of WBV for neurological and other health issues needs more research. But this hypothesis fits my experiences with myself and my clients. It also might explain in part why my clients' results are generally significantly better than reported in the scientific literature since much of the current research is based on results using asynchronous (double motor) machines or other machines I do not recommend. In summary, given my personal experience and results with clients, I only recommend the fully synchronized vibration that results from a single motor vibration machine.

Whole body vibration has many wonderful benefits, but the issue of brain synchronization and optimal brain functioning is critical to long-term benefits and health, including, I suspect, optimal long-term muscle strength and athletic ability. My machines are designed to give you optimal conditioning for the whole body, including the brain.

Does Whole Body Vibration Work Like Meditation?

In recent years, there has been a surge of interest in meditation as an aid in healing. Science and medicine have shown meditation's effectiveness in improving mental and physical health. Over 3,000 studies on mindfulness meditation have shown that it can improve sleep, help you lose weight, lower stress levels, decrease loneliness in seniors, improve attention, manage chronic pain, reduce stress and depression, treat binge eating and other eating disorders, and contribute to greater cell longevity. An important aspect of mindfulness meditation is to focus your attention on your body and be in the present moment—things that WBV is very good at helping you do. Almost automatically, you will begin to do so as the vibration floods through your body.

WBV has not been studied as an aid to meditation, but logically and intuitively this idea makes sense. WBV is such a powerful physical sensation throughout every part of your body that it almost forces you to pay attention to your body if you are not distracting yourself by watching TV or some other activity. Focusing your thoughts on your body connects your mind to your body and brings the mind into the present moment as opposed to worrying about the many things we all find to obsess and worry about, in a similar way to mindfulness meditation.

Brain entrainment methods such as sound recordings and other repetitive calming stimuli are also commonly used to help people meditate. If WBV is a form of brain entrainment—synching our brain waves—then perhaps WBV is also slowing our brain waves down as seen with meditation. Perhaps WBV is helping our brains move to a meditative state as a guiding force in WBV's healing effect. Research in this area, including mapping brain wave states while using WBV, could be enlightening.

In more than two decades of using WBV, I have had many people report that they almost immediately feel more alive, awake, and rejuvenated in their minds. They report suddenly tackling a project that seemed too difficult before (like writing reports and papers or, in my case, books) and having improvements in mood, focus, concentration, and even memory. I am excited by the possibilities and plan to pursue research in this area as soon as possible.

Could You Use Some Brain Stimulation?

Are you reaching your potential? Who even knows what their potential is? I believe it is usually much greater than we realize, but life, poor health, environmental factors, and our own negative thinking get in our way. In addition, beginning in their late twenties, most people will lose about 1 percent annually of the cells in the hippocampus, a key portion of the brain related to memory and certain types of learning. And since the brain is connected to all parts of the body, almost all health issues—especially depression, anxiety, memory loss, low energy, and nervous system diseases—will improve with a better functioning brain. Give yourself the gift of whole body vibration, and your brain will repay you with opportunities you cannot yet even imagine.

Chapter 5

Boost Your Energy

Energy and Your Life

Busy, busy, busy . . . so much to do and so little time. For many people, modern life has become a race where time is a scarce and precious commodity. Others have been running so hard and are so stressed that they have become chronically fatigued and can barely move anymore. But what if you could boost your physical energy level, balance and focus your mind, and raise your spiritual energy all at the same time? What might that do for you and for your ability to accomplish your goals, find your true path, and enjoy your life?

On the physical level, there are several energy-increasing effects that have been demonstrated with the use of WBV. Research has shown that increases in testosterone levels are linked to greater energy for men and women, as well as heightened libido and sexual performance[102] (see Chapter 7). Circulation also improves, which provides more nutrients and oxygen to all cells, thus producing energy. As the exercise and workouts increase muscle strength, so the whole body gains power and strength.

In the brain, WBV causes levels of the neurotransmitter serotonin to increase rapidly. High levels of serotonin improve sleep and promote a relaxed, happy, confident state of mind in which people are likely to be more active. Nothing saps your energy like depression and exhaustion, which can make just getting out of bed seem impossible.

WBV also works on the electromagnetic level. Every time you are on a vibration plate, all your neurons are activated, shooting electromagnetic energy through your body and brain. This electromagnetic energy is fundamentally connected to our physical and mental states. Norman Shealy, MD, PhD, founder of the American Holistic Medical Association and world-famous neurosurgeon, discusses this connection in his 2006 book *Soul Medicine*. "The body's electromagnetic field," Shealy writes, "is a means through which biochemistry and physical anatomy interact with unseen energies. . . . In its component parts, and in its aggregate whole, our bodies, souls, minds, and emotional realms are interrelated energy systems. Energetic treatment of one part of this living matrix always affects the whole."[103]

TESTIMONIALS

When I first started vibration therapy, I was so chronically fatigued that I would get a cart at the supermarket to lean on while I walked around, even if I only needed one item. After every vibration session (two per week), I felt stronger and energized; I was noticeably gaining vigor by the week. Two months into the therapy, there was a snowstorm that dropped a half a foot of snow overnight. I was late to my vibration appointment that day because first I had to shovel out my driveway, and then I shoveled out my neighbor's driveway as she is frail and elderly.

—Ellen Lehn, 57 years old

I had been vibrating just a few times when I went home after my three or four minutes of vibration, and I had so much energy I started scrubbing the kitchen floor by hand. When I finished with the floor, I started in on the walls. My husband, who was half asleep on the couch where we would usually both be after a long day at work, said to me, "What has gotten into you?"

—Marianne L., age 50+

Life Force or Chi Energy

Western medicine recognizes that the nervous system is a pattern of electromagnetic signals. An EEG measures electronic brain waves, and an MRI creates images of the brain by measuring its electromagnetic energy. Quantum physics describes the world of subatomic particles that make up all matter and from which electromagnetic energy arises. Quantum physicist Ervin Lazlo explains that science is in the midst of a "shift from matter to energy as the primary reality. . . . There is no categorical divide between the physical world, the living world, and the world of mind and consciousness."[104] Shealy describes the quantum universe as "a set of probabilities, susceptible to influence by many factors, including thought, will, and intention."[105]

Many cultures throughout time have recognized the existence of a life-force energy. The Chinese call it chi, Indians call it prana, and European traditions have called it life force, soul, spirit, vital energy, vital principle, elan, and more. This energy guides and powers a person's body and life, and disturbances in this energy due to trauma of any sort can have a profound effect on your physical and mental state.

Thousands of years ago, the Chinese discovered and mapped "energy meridians" in the body. Each of these energy pathways is associated with different organs and bodily systems. The Chinese medical system of acupuncture is based on maintaining a healthy and balanced flow of energy in those different meridians. Indian medicine describes chakras, spinning energy vortexes in our bodies, also associated with particular body systems and organs. In fact, some people can sense their own vibrational energy, and when these people stand on a vibrating plate, they report feeling energy shooting through their energy meridians and their chakras unblocking and spinning faster.

There is, in fact, measurable electromagnetic energy emanating from all things because all substances are made from molecules that are, in turn, made from even smaller vibrating particles that have positive or negative electrical charges. Thus, every substance has an electromagnetic charge that can be measured with sensitive scientific equipment. For example, Kirlian photography can detect and record the electromagnetic wavelengths around a person or object.[106]

Another energy measuring system that medical doctors in Europe use frequently is "electrodermal testing," developed in the 1950s. It is a computer-linked testing system in which a probe that detects electromagnetic energy is touched to different acupuncture points on the hands and feet, and the energy in the associated energy meridian is graphed on a computer screen.[107] With this system, you can instantly see which energy meridians and thus their associated body organs or systems are in balance, stressed (too much energy), or weakened (too little energy).

There are more than 100,000 such electrodermal screening machines in use worldwide, although there are very few in the United States where acceptance of energy medicine has been limited. There are many accounts of the detection of diseases, allergies, and toxic states using these machines.[108] Before spending a lot of time and money, we can see which therapies or products resonate with an individual's electromagnetic energy and are therefore most likely to be successful. Electrodermal testing will also register changes in energy before and after vibration. I have seen this many times in my natural health practice where I regularly use both vibration and electrodermal testing.

Piezoelectricity?

On the physical level, WBV stimulates electromagnetic energy through a physical property of crystals called piezoelectricity—the ability of crystals to turn mechanical vibration into electrical vibration. Our bodies are living liquid crystals in the sense that we are highly organized molecular structures, and as such, we have the property of piezoelectricity. Dr. Norman Shealy describes our "bodies, souls, minds, and emotional realm" as a "living matrix" with the property of piezoelectricity.[109] "Waves of mechanical vibration moving through the living matrix produce electrical fields and vice versa. . . . Connective tissue is a liquid crystalline semiconductor. Piezoelectric signals from the cells can travel throughout the body in this medium."[110] The result is that "energetic treatment of one part of this living matrix always affects the whole."[111]

Thus, every time you are on a vibration plate, your neurons fire, shooting electromagnetic energy through your body and brain as

Every time you are on a vibration plate, your neurons fire, shooting electromagnetic energy through your body and brain . . . to heal, balance, and unblock your energy systems. your body turns the mechanical vibration into the electrical energy vibrations you need to heal, balance, and unblock your energy systems. Energy will flow into and through your energy meridians and chakra energy centers, increasing their proper spinning and energy flow. Since these energy meridians and chakras are also linked to different organs, body systems, emotions and needs, improving the flow of energy will help heal the physical body and mind, and improve life— all at the same time.

Pain Management through Electromagnetic Energy?

There are often rapid and dramatic decreases in pain for people who use WBV, as is also commonly seen with energy medicine.[112,113,114,115] Acupuncture is one of the more familiar of these methods in the United States. Dr. Shealy, one of the early gurus of alternative health and a groundbreaking innovator in energy medicine, reports marked improvement using acupuncture in 70 percent of people with rheumatoid arthritis who failed to improve with conventional medicine; 75 percent of people with migraines; 80 percent of people with diabetic neuropathy; 70 percent of people with depression; and 70 percent of people with chronic low back pain.[116]

In China, where acupuncture originated, surgeries are sometimes performed with only the aid of acupuncture. That is hard to believe, but I can say from personal experience that acupuncture does have a remarkable ability to control pain. I am very pain sensitive, usually requiring extra Novocain for the slightest dental procedure, but I once had a tooth pulled using only acupuncture during a period when I could not tolerate any Western medicine drugs. Gripping the dental chair in fear, to my amazement I

WBV is like acupuncture in its ability to stimulate our electromagnetic system.

only felt a wrenching, pulling sensation—no pain. WBV is like acupuncture in its ability to stimulate our electromagnetic system, and I have seen hundreds of people step on a whole body vibration plate only to get off one to two minutes later with their pain gone. The placebo effect is unlikely in this situation since this often happens with people who have never heard of this possibility. It has happened at crowded expos where I didn't have time to mention it to people who had never heard of WBV.

TESTIMONIAL

I have struggled for years with chronic fatigue. After each WBV session (just standing on the plate for a few minutes) I am amazed at the energy I got, energy I haven't had for years. And I found that I could focus on tasks that I had been struggling with. After the first once-a-week session, my energy lasted for a day or two. The morning after the second session, I jumped out of bed for the first time in about twenty years, plus my mind was clear and focused. By the fifth session, my energy lasted for an entire week. I'm so glad I took Becky Chambers' class – I love the way I feel.

—Peg MacNeil

TESTIMONIAL

I met Becky Chambers when I was in my late 60s. Up to that time I exercised 3-4 times per week at a local gym, ate a mostly healthy diet, and maintained a regular weight. However, my energy felt stuck in survival, and anxiety was taking over. I was experiencing fatigue and unexplained health issues. A bone density test result was not good even though I followed the doctor's advice. I needed to find out how to turn this around in a natural way. I needed to get my energy unstuck so that I could heal.

I started working with Becky and WBV in October 2019. The difference in how I felt was almost immediate – physically and emotionally. Within a week, I felt emotions such as fear and anxiety over my health, finances, and survival begin to surface and release. As I continued with the WBV, my focus sharpened, my energy and faith grew stronger, and negative emotions moved out and dissipated at a faster pace, sometimes within hours, and eventually within minutes. Simultaneously my body was becoming stronger, more vibrant. Energy was moving. Healing was accelerating on multiple levels.

A few months later, when the 2020 pandemic hit, everyone in my office was sent home to work, the gym was closed, isolation ensued, and the news reports were not good. And yet I was happy. I focused on the good.

I do WBV twenty minutes most days. My muscles are stronger, and my emotional well-being is consistently positive and happy. The anxiety is a distant memory. WBV and energy-focused counseling with Becky Chambers are a huge factor in changing the quality of my life for the better.

I want to thank Becky for her never-ending search for healing on every level and her commitment to sharing her expertise.

—Debra Dahlman, late 60s

Chapter 6

Pain Relief

With pain being a major quality of life factor for millions of people and dependence on pain-killing drugs leading to further health issues, the capacity to reduce pain is a life-changing benefit of whole body vibration (WBV).

There are numerous pathways through which WBV can relieve pain, including lowering inflammation, relaxing tight muscles, lowering stress and anxiety, and an acupuncture-like pain-reducing effect[ii] (also see Chapter 5).

WBV has been shown to reduce inflammation (see Chapter 2), and when there are nerves in an area of inflammation, there will also be pain. As a 2021 scientific review of pain management noted, "Pain is a consequential phenomenon of inflammatory responses."[117] WBV also balances gut flora and calms gut inflammation, which can directly alleviate digestive system distress, and since gut health is linked to inflammation levels in general, it can potentially relieve pain throughout the body.

Certain types of pain relief from WBV, including back pain and fi-

---

ii   Acupuncture is quite well accepted at this point as an effective treatment for pain. It is even covered by many health insurance companies, although exactly how acupunture lowers pain has not been clearly established.

bromyalgia, are thought to be linked to WBV's powerful muscle relaxing and stretching effects. Even if you are just standing on the plate, WBV is working like a massage as it strengthens your muscles, loosens tight muscles and connective tissue, and strengthens muscle fibers.

Stress reduction and mental health effects are another mode of pain relief. According to Harvard Medical School, "Pain is depressing, and depression causes and intensifies pain"[118] for many types of pain, including headaches, backaches, arthritis, and chronic pain conditions such as fibromyalgia. As we saw in the last chapter, WBV can relieve depression and anxiety, giving it yet another pathway for reducing pain.

Whether you know exactly how WBV is reducing your pain or not, that won't stop you from enjoying the relief.

Scientific Research on WBV and Pain

Research has shown clear evidence that some types of pain such as chronic lower back pain, muscle pain, fibromyalgia, diabetic neuropathy, and knee pain from osteoarthritis decrease with WBV.

For example, a 2019 study of forty-two men with nonspecific low back pain concluded that "pain was significantly reduced after 12-week WBV exercise in NSLBP [nonspecific low back pain] patients."[119] Another study in 2017 of lower back pain among working people in Scandinavia concluded that "WBV training seems to be an effective, safe, and suitable intervention for seated working employees with chronic low-back pain."[120]

Two other studies gave early indications of the benefits of WBV for back pain. A 2002 study with sixty

Back Pain

"Interestingly, well-controlled vibration may be the cure rather than the cause of lower back pain."

subjects concluded, "Interestingly, well-controlled vibration may be the cure rather than the cause of lower back pain."[121] Another study concluded that WBV "may represent a novel physical therapy for patients with non-specific low back pain."[122]

Early research showed evidence that WBV can create muscle relaxation, potentially reducing muscle pain. Promising results with young people both stimulated musculoskeletal activity and an immediate increase in musculoskeletal relaxation.[123] This research gave hope that WBV could be used for more complex musculoskeletal disorders such as fibromyalgia.

TESTIMONIAL

Becky, I have to say thank you! I had been going to physical therapy for four months, multiple times a week for my right hip. I do have some arthritis in both hips, but my issue was muscle related. We'd get the two sets of muscles to relax and be fine for 2–3 days before they would tighten up again. I was doing my stretches multiple times a day, and we hit a plateau. I decided to stop PT and see how I did with only the stretches. While at my monthly massage, the therapist asked if I heard of WBV. Recently some of her clients told her about WBV and the success they were having. I went home and ordered your Power 1000. After four days of 1 minute sessions, the pain went from 9–10 to zero! I've continued to use it 5–6 times a week. I'll never stop using it, and I recommend it to everyone.

—Debbie Larson

Indeed, WBV research on fibromyalgia with middle-aged women has shown potential to relieve pain and improve quality of life. A 2017 survey of four studies on fibromyalgia with a total of 150 middle-aged women reported, "Two studies compared WBV combined with mixed exercise versus control and found evidence of positive effects on HRQL [health-related quality of life], pain intensity, fatigue, stiffness, and strength."[124] The results were strong enough for the authors to write that there was "evidence of positive effects on HRQL, pain intensity, fatigue, stiffness, and strength."[125] But due to the low sample size of the individual studies and other study quality issues, further research was recommended to determine the best method for WBV use with fibromyalgia.

Fibromyalgia

There was "evidence of positive effects on HRQL, pain intensity, fatigue, stiffness, and strength."

Peripheral Neuropathy

"WBV improves sensory sensations like pain and vibration perception, neuropathy disability score, balance measures and health-related QOL [quality of life] in PDPN [painful diabetic peripheral neuropathy]."

Research on peripheral nerve pain and disability, particularly as a result of diabetic neuropathy, has also yielded promising results. In one 2020 study of twenty participants where approximately half in a control group were given a sham vibration (sound without motion), a significant pain reduction was seen at both two and four weeks after the WBV began. WBV also alleviated pain for up to six weeks after the WBV was stopped.[126]

A second peripheral neuropathy

study, also published in 2020, yielded similar results. This study of twenty-six men and women in their fifties and sixties also had a control group that did not receive WBV.[127] The conclusion in this study was also that WBV was successful in improving peripheral neuropathy. "WBV improves sensory sensations like pain and vibration perception, neuropathy disability score, balance measures and health-related QOL [quality of life] in PDPN [painful diabetic peripheral neuropathy]."[128]

TESTIMONIALS

I have really enjoyed the vibrating foot massager for my peripheral neuropathy. I have had diabetes Type 1 for over thirty-five years with peripheral neuropathy for the last two years. I recently started using the foot vibrator and rapidly began to notice an improvement. My peripheral neuropathy is not painful, but there is numbness, or a lack of sensation – it feels like I'm wearing slippers. The vibration restores my sensation. Thank you, Becky Chambers!

—A. DeBord, MD, retired

When I first started working with Becky Chambers about three months ago, I had constant pain in my right hip, right thigh, and both knees. I frequently walked with a limp, and climbing stairs was excruciatingly painful. In the last three months, I have made dramatic improvements. I was able to return to moderate exercising, and I have no pain in my hips or thighs. If anyone had told me that I could be so much stronger or that my pain could be reduced so much in such a brief period of time, I never would have believed it.

—Ann MacGibbon, PhD, age 58

Knee Osteoarthritis

"WBV combined with exercise was superior to exercise alone, in improving pain, physical function (TUG test and WOMAC), and knee extensor strength."

The effectiveness of WBV for some kinds of pain such as knee osteoarthritis (KOA) has been controversial. After years of sometimes confusing results, the latest large 2022 meta-analysis research study on osteoarthritis knee pain has found clear and encouraging results. Citing a larger pool of studies and trial size, researchers concluded that WBV is a safe and effective training method for knee osteoarthritis and more effective than conventional exercise in some measures. "WBV combined with exercise was superior to exercise alone, in improving pain, physical function (TUG test and WOMAC), and knee extensor strength."[129] However, the authors do note that the evidence remains controversial, and there remains a need for more research to determine optimal regimens.

TESTIMONIAL

I am a fifty-seven-year-old tradesman. After a lifetime of hard physical work, I had come to expect arthritic pain as a normal part of my workday. My ankles, knees, hips, and lower back jabbed at me constantly, and my response had been to tough it out. It was a losing proposition, and it appeared that hip replacement was inevitable.

When a friend offered to let me try her vibration machine, the skeptic in me thought, "yeah, right." That was weeks ago. This morning, I scampered down the stairs like a teenager. The remarkable thing is that I felt relief after the first five-minute session. Now, I simply stand on my WBV machine for five minutes each morning and head off to work with a happy song in my heart. The pain has gone. Imagine that.

—Wayne Young, master electrician, age 57

Conflicting Results

Earlier knee osteoarthritis research has been confusing with some research concluding that WBV improves knee osteoarthritis pain[130,131,132] and others concluding that it does not.[133,134,135] For example, in an earlier 2015 systematic review of WBV's effects on knee arthritis,[136] the combined data showed statistically significant improvement in knee pain and function. But individually, only two of the five studies in that meta-analysis concluded that knee pain was reduced.[137]

What accounts for the conflicting results? I believe the answer may be similar to the issue regarding neurological diseases and other chronic health issues with WBV. Success may lie in how and what type of WBV is used, especially with more fragile populations such as older people and those with health issues.

My Research Survey Results

When the correct type of vibration is used and my guidelines for a slow and gentle approach are followed, I have had clearly positive results for pain reduction in older people.

My own research survey[138] of fifty-three of my customers (out of 187 surveys sent) reported large gains in pain reduction. Our respondents reported an average 31 percent drop in pain levels of many types (over one-third reporting knee pain reduction), with 74 percent of those in pain reporting a 52 percent drop in their pain levels (see Appendix 1 for a summary of the survey methods and results). This is particularly significant because 90 percent of my customers and clients are over the age of fifty, and older people with health issues are a population in which good results with WBV are harder to obtain. Further research to confirm my results using more rigorous research methodology is currently underway, but as a preliminary study, the results are encouraging.

Using the Vibrant Health Power 1000 vibration machine, 74 percent of those in pain reported a 52 percent drop in their pain level.

While not every person in my survey reported a reduction in pain, some people reported nearly complete disappearances of pain within weeks of beginning WBV. For all those in pain, the overall average pain reduction was 31 percent. This survey covered many different types and locations of pain—back pain, joint pain, muscle pain, and nerve pain.

The changes were also sometimes very rapid, even immediately after one session or within a few WBV sessions, clearly pointing to WBV and not some other unaccounted-for factor as responsible for the reported changes. Such rapid reductions in pain and inflammation may be evidence of WBV's effects on the electromagnetic system since they happen too fast to attribute them to other causes.

Like exercise, the ideal way to use WBV for continued lifelong health is to incorporate WBV into your life as part of your daily routine. This is easy to do since it is quick, feels great, and supplies instant gratification as well as long-term benefits.

To achieve lasting pain reduction, however, most people require regular sessions (usually two to three times per week) for at least a couple of months. Like exercise, the ideal way to use WBV for continued lifelong health is to incorporate WBV into your life as part of your daily routine. This is easy to do since it is quick, feels great, and supplies instant gratification as well as long-term benefits. I do, however, recommend adding other natural health methods to your WBV program because they can work synergistically, leading to greater effects.

OPIOID ADDICTION

WBV may even possibly be of use in the fight against opioid addiction, in particular by helping people avoid becoming addicted in the first place. While WBV is not recommended for immediate use after acute injuries or procedures and cannot replace powerful opioids, WBV is an effective natural system to lower pain without the use of drugs. WBV also raises serotonin, norepinephrine, and testosterone, which can give people the boost to mood and energy they often seek from opioids. With the aid of these effects, WBV may be helpful in weaning people off of or possibly avoiding entirely addictive pain killers for chronic conditions, thus avoiding addiction. For example, in my research survey, some of the people reporting pain reduction were also reducing the amount of their pain medication or switching to a less powerful pain medication at the same time.

TESTIMONIAL

In 2008, according to the medical professionals, I needed both shoulders replaced. I was in a great deal of pain for years and was unable to raise my arms to reach anything above my head due to the pain and joint limitations. I had to modify all my exercise and drop cross-country skiing, mountain climbing, and yoga because of the pain and limited use of my shoulders and upper body. Depression from this limiting situation had me crying many days as exercise and wellness had always been a huge part of my life. The pain was intense, twenty-four hours a day.

My vibration machine, in combination with eating well and an exercise program of rebounding, walking, and doing the elliptical four to five times a week, has been a huge factor in lessening the twenty-four-hour pain I had in both shoulders. The shoulders still need replacing, but because the pain is not bothering me, I can postpone the medical procedure.

—Wendy MacLean, small business co-owner

Why are Vibrant Health's results better than other research results? In a nutshell, I believe most researchers are using too much vibration and the wrong type of machine so the intensity of the vibration experience is too great. They are more focused on increasing muscle strength without taking into account the need to calm the brain and body. Too powerful of a vibration experience and/or the use of the wrong machine might also send an asynchronous signal into the brain (see "My Experience with Desynchronization" in Chapter 4)—the opposite of a calming, destressing experience that is most effective for healing. These two factors—intensity and quality—are critical. When they are not correct, WBV can create too much stress for the body and mind, leading to poor results.

WBV is much more than just a workout. It affects every part of your body, including your brain and

WBV is much more than just a workout. It affects every part of your body, including your brain and nervous system. As your brain is guiding your internal health and well-being along with the rest of your life, it is critical to use vibration that is calming and synchronizing.

nervous system. As your brain is guiding your internal health and well-being along with the rest of your life, it is critical to use vibration that is calming and synchronizing.

Researchers, WBV companies, and consumers don't realize how powerful WBV really is. WBV was originally developed for Olympic athletes, and it is still best known, marketed, and sold for its intense workout effect. Because of this tunnel-vision bias where increased muscle strength is the expected and primary goal of WBV, researchers use machines that are too powerful and not carefully designed for the smooth, synchronized vibration that may be best for your brain, and they try to do too much WBV too soon.

Vibrant Health machines provide vibration that can be adjusted to the sweet spot for you as you heal and become stronger. They provide a smooth, purely synchronized vibration with an amplitude, g-force, and frequency range that creates just the right degree of intensity that is effective but not too stressful. With a careful program of use while following my guidelines, rapid pain relief is the result for most people.

Chapter 7

Rejuvenation: Sex, Beauty, and Mobility

Feeling the Pain . . .

Oh my achin' joints!

Getting old is no picnic! Sex loses its appeal, beauty becomes an expensive full-time project, and mobility is a creaky, painful exercise of adjusting to limitations. But perhaps the fountain of youth does exist—and it vibrates! WBV has numerous global rejuvenation effects such as increasing stem cells levels,[139] raising human growth hormone (HGH) and testosterone,[140] increasing circulation to all cells, detoxification, muscle and nerve stimulation, and energy balancing. These effects help your body repair its tissues and functions, and the effects can be especially dramatic with sexual libido and performance; skin tone and color; body shape; cellulite and fat deposits; and joint flexibility, pain, and strength.

Consider the case of cats. Cats have "nine lives" . . . and they purr—essentially a built-in whole body vibration system. Cats purr, or vibrate, when they are happy but also when they are sick or stressed. Cats generally have strong bones and joint health throughout most of their lives, allowing them to survive falls that no other animal can. Researchers who looked at the records of 132 cat falls from an average height of five and a half stories found that 90 percent had survived. The record height for a cat falling and surviving is forty-five stories. They have an amazing ability to heal injured bones, muscles, tendons, ligaments, and joints; and they can usually bounce back rapidly from other illnesses. Is purring the root of the myth that cats have nine lives? (Lev G. Fedyniak, "Can Your Cat's Purr Heal?" Animal Wellness, September 12, 2010, https://animalwellnessmagazine.com/cats-purr-heal/.)

Stem Cells

Stem cells are the holy grail of repair and regeneration of the body. These cells are unique in their ability to develop into many different types of cells and thus regenerate tissues and organs throughout the body. They are considered "the origin of the growth and development of human beings" with "huge potential benefit in disease treatment"[141] because stem cells have the potential to develop into specialized cells as varied as muscle, blood, and brain cells. Stem cell therapies, sometimes using complicated procedures to harvest these cells from one part of your body and inject them into another area and sometimes using drugs, have so far been used to treat over 100 different diseases. Now it appears that you can gain the regenerative powers of stem cell treatment with greater safety and ease just by standing on your vibration machine.

The same research study by the U.S. Military in 2022 that found greater inflammation improvements with WBV than with exercise also found circulating stem cell levels to be superior with WBV.[142]

While exercise is known to increase stem cells, WBV has been found to increase stem cells to a greater degree. The highest levels of stem cells and other regenerative growth factors were seen with the use of WBV plus exercise, so for the best results, don't forget your regular aerobic exercise. WBV plus exercise led to a 39 percent increase in circulating stem cells, a 33 percent increase with WBV alone, and a 21 percent increase with exercise only.

Stem cells are unique in their ability to develop into many different types of cells and thus regenerate tissues and organs all over the body. WBV plus exercise led to a 39 percent increase in circulating stem cells, a 33 percent increase with WBV alone, and a 21 percent increase with exercise only.

Human Growth Hormone

Another important benefit of WBV is increased levels of human growth hormone (HGH), which promotes the healing of tissues critical for joint health and mobility (ligaments, tendons, muscles, bones, and nerves) along with all other tis-

Another important benefit of WBV is increased levels of HGH, which promotes the healing and rejuvenation of all tissues.

sues. HGH levels typically fall with age, and any method of raising them is hotly pursued by those interested in rejuvenation of any sort, whether it is for athletic performance, daily pain relief and function, sexual libido and function, or beauty.

Early research (2000) showed promising results with WBV, increasing HGH levels up to 150 percent.[143,144,145,146] Several recent studies have since confirmed increases of HGH with WBV.[147,148,149]

Testosterone

WBV has been shown to increase levels of the sex hormone testosterone.[150,151,152,153,154] Normally, as men get older, their testosterone levels gradually decline—typically by about 1 percent per year after age thirty. Women have testosterone levels about 10 percent of men's to begin with, and their testosterone levels drop rapidly at menopause. Testosterone, the major sex hormone for males, is closely linked to libido and sexual performance in men, as well as overall energy levels. Testosterone is also important for women.

WBV has been shown to increase levels of the sex hormone testosterone. . . . Testosterone, the major sex hormone for males, is closely linked to libido and sexual performance . . . , [and it] is also important for women.

Psychiatrist Susan Rako wrote a groundbreaking book in 1996 called *The Hormone of Desire: The Truth about Testosterone, Sexuality, and Menopause* (updated in 1999), which is still in print and still the most comprehensive and accurate body of information about the physiology and function of testosterone in women's bodies. In her book, Dr.

Rako describes her experience and the research that has shown that testosterone levels affect libido (meaning one's "life force," not just sexual drive) for both men and women. In Dr. Rako's words, testosterone is "essential . . . to the healthy functioning of virtually all tissues in her [a woman's] body, and to her experience of vital energy and sexual libido."[155] Typical high-testosterone qualities include focused motivation, assertiveness, a sense of power, and enhanced sex drive. Healthy levels of testosterone help women take risks and live their lives with exuberance.

Testosterone also has powerful anti-aging effects. It turns fat into muscle, keeps skin supple, increases bone mineral density, gives us a positive mood, and boosts our ability to handle stress. It supports mental health and cognitive functioning, as well as liver function and blood vessel health. Low testosterone levels have been associated with heart attack, Alzheimer's disease, osteoporosis, and depression.

Testosterone is "essential . . . to the healthy functioning of virtually all tissues in [a woman's] body and to her experience of vital energy and sexual libido."

There are drugs, including Androgel, that are designed to raise testosterone in men, but as is generally true with prescription drugs, there are side effects,[156] and women and children must carefully avoid contact with these gels or their hormone balances may be thrown off. The list of common side effects for men include nausea, vomiting, headache, dizziness, hair loss, trouble sleeping, change in sexual desire, redness or swelling of the skin, change in skin color, and acne.

Side effects that are unlikely but serious include breast pain or enlargement; swelling of feet and ankles; weight gain; very slow, shallow, difficult breathing; and weakness. Rare but very serious side effects include trouble urinating, mental or mood changes (e.g., depression, agitation, hostility), change in size or shape of the testicles, testicular pain or tenderness, stomach or abdominal pain, dark urine, change in the amount of urine, yellowing of eyes or skin, calf tenderness, swelling, or pain. Why risk all this when there is a safe, natural approach that has many positive "side effects"?

While testosterone in the form of gels, creams, or pills is sometimes prescribed for women, the long-term safety of testosterone drug therapy for women is unknown. At this time, no commonly prescribed testosterone preparations have been approved by the Food and Drug Administration for use in women. If a testosterone drug is prescribed for women, it is off-label and not tested for safety.

WBV will neither raise testosterone levels too high or too fast nor interact negatively with other drugs or bodily functions. WBV promotes the body's ability to achieve its highest natural state of health. This is not to say that WBV is totally without risk. There are contraindications (see Appendix 2), and it is important to understand detoxification and nutrition, but as a natural therapy, WBV promotes the optimal natural functioning of all body organs and systems.

Other WBV Effects That Improve Libido and Sex

WBV also raises serotonin (see Chapter 4), a neurotransmitter in the brain that is important for mood and the ability to experience pleasure, including sexual pleasure. Confidence and a good mood go a long way toward improving sexual experiences. The increase in strength and physical energy levels associated with WBV will also help with sexual performance.

Another critical area affecting sexuality is your chi energy. Because of the piezoelectrical ability of the human body that converts mechanical vibration into electromagnetic energy (see Chapter 5), every time you are on a vibration plate you will be sending energy through the entire chakra system. All that energy will first pass through the Kundalini chakra—the seat of your most basic survival needs, including sexual energy.

People who are sensitive to this energy can sometimes actually feel their chakras spinning. When these people stand on a vibrating plate, their eyes glaze over with delight, and they talk about feeling energy shooting through meridians and chakras unblocking and spinning faster.

Whether people can identify "energy" or not, I have had some humorous situations develop when people try the Body Vibe machines at expos. Some people end up suddenly feeling *very good indeed,* and the more uninhibited ones are not shy about expressing themselves. Strangers up and down the aisles turn to see what all the excitement, laughing, and oohs and aahs are about. Since this happens even with very gentle Body Vibe models on which you cannot physically feel the vibration past your knees, and since it happens quickly (in thirty to sixty seconds), it seems that at least some of this reaction is due to electromagnetic energy transmitting through the body rather than hormonal or direct physical stimulation.

My favorite story of increasing libido and sexual enjoyment involves a middle-aged woman who came to me twice a week for three weeks. She was primarily interested in losing weight and increasing bone density. Her husband, though, who was quite skeptical, said, "So, you think you are going to lose weight and increase bone density just by standing on that machine?" But after three weeks, my client came to me and said, "I think those hormonal effects you were talking about might be kicking in. Now my husband says, '*Buy one!*'"

TESTIMONIAL

I didn't need to lose weight, but with WBV I am firmer, and pants are looser. I need a belt now. Libido has also increased, getting ready to date again after three years alone.

—Dave H. age 68

Beauty

Beauty is mostly health and happiness radiating through our bodies. Since WBV is fantastic for your physical and emotional health, you will be beautiful too. Working out on your Body Vibe will tone your body, balance hormones, increase neurotransmitters in your brain, help you lose fat and cellulite, increase circulation to all tissues (resulting in increased collagen production which tightens and smoothes skin), and put color in your cheeks and a sparkle in your eyes. When you feel good, you take better care of yourself by eating wisely, exercising more, maybe even sprucing up your wardrobe and changing your hair style. Then you get promoted at work because you're more effective and radiating confidence. It's like a snowball rolling downhill—it just keeps getting bigger and better all the time.

While cellulite and wrinkles are normal signs of aging, with improved health they can be delayed or decreased. Cellulite is the lumpy appearance of fat that develops primarily in women, much to their annoyance, especially on the thighs, knees, backside, and upper arms. But cellulite is not really a fat problem and has nothing to do with how much you weigh. Cellulite is made of a special type of fat called subcutaneous that is within the skin layer. It can't be burned as fuel, so you don't lose it by dieting.

As we age, circulation begins to decrease (especially to the thighs and other cellulite-prone areas) due to blood vessel damage and the effects of decreasing estrogen. Poor circulation leads to a lack of nutrients and more toxins building up in the skin, which further damages blood vessels and lowers collagen production (the major component of a connective-tissue support structure that holds the subcutaneous fat in place). This all means that fat bulges out through the spaces between the fibers of that collagen support structure, creating the lumpy effect. In other words, as one doctor put it, your backside is something like an old mattress with the stuffing bulging out.

Wrinkles are due to the loss of subcutaneous fat that, together with a healthy connective-tissue structure, usually plumps out and smoothes skin. They are also due to the loss of elastin, which gives skin its flexibility and allows it to stretch and give without damage.

WBV increases circulation, thus attacking the root cause of cellulite and wrinkles.

WBV increases circulation, thus attacking the root cause of cellulite and wrinkles. Increased circulation brings more nutrients to the skin, causing greater collagen production, which strengthens the connective-tissue structure, holding that unruly subcutaneous fat in place. Meanwhile, those nasty toxins and their associated free-radical damage are flushed out, further helping your skin glow and retain its youthful appearance. WBV also increases HGH, which promotes the healing of all tissues, including connective tissue and skin cells. Hop on a vibration machine, and you are fighting the "do not go gently into that good night" battle on all fronts.

Add good nutrition and nutritional supplements, and you have fresh troops pouring over the hills laden with supplies. Protein sources contain keratin, a building block for collagen and elastin, and antioxidants (fruits and vegetables) neutralize free-radical damage from toxins. Anti-aging creams are available now with these very ingredients incorporated into them, but keep in mind that nutrients are much more effectively absorbed into cells from the bloodstream than through the skin.

Also, be sure to get plenty of potassium (all fruits) but low sodium to maintain the proper electrolyte balance that promotes hydration of your cells. Get lots of omega-3 oils to keep blood vessels and cell walls healthy. Together, these two factors ensure good hydration to your cells—again, a much more effective approach than hydrating the skin with lotions. Of course, you can always do both—lotions and nutrition—but don't forget the healthy food. As your mother said, "Eat your vegetables!"

TESTIMONIALS

Going on the vibration plate feels like a mini vacation. I enjoy it, it relaxes me, and my body feels happy. At night, the body pain I had in bed is gone, and there is a real satisfaction in my sleeping that I have not had for years. I am more in tune and listening to my body, and I have much more courage and the willpower to start a physical activity like biking. This feels very en-couraging, and I am excited to see how my health continues to improve.

I have also noticed that the varicose veins on my legs are getting much better. They have stopped bulging out and seem to be slowly fading away. This is excit-ing as I was not expecting to improve this issue with the vibration. I feel like so many options are opening to me, with a future that I was not expecting. Thank you so much, Becky Chambers!

—Giuseppe Pallotta, age 52

In the fall of 2020, my bone density results came back, and I was once again in the osteopenia category after reversing it four years prior. Not wanting to take medications, I asked my osteopath what other options I had. She mentioned the Whole Body Vibrator as one of my options.

Each time I visited my osteopath after that, she was impressed with the fluidity in my previously rigid back. After a while I realized that all my pain was gone—after having had scoliosis and muscle spasms for many years—and I felt more energetic.

I am now pain free for the first time in many years, sleeping more soundly, and enjoying renewed energy. On top of that, I even look better than I did in photos from 20 years ago!

I recommend this wonderful machine as an integral part of your wellness routine. Just 10 minutes a day makes a world of difference. But I warn you, take it slow as Becky Chambers so aptly stresses, and you will soon be enjoying better health and vitality!

Gratefully,

—Mary Lincoln Brown, age 74

Mobility

One of the most well-known and accepted uses of WBV is for physical therapy. Entire books have been written about it.[157] It is used in physical therapy centers around the world. Sports franchises and top athletes use WBV for athletic training and to help athletes heal faster from injuries, and they are less likely to be injured in the first place because their joints are stronger.

WBV is effective therapy for a wide range of joint and movement issues, including arthritis, bursitis, tendonitis, pulled and strained muscles, weakness, range of motion issues, poor flexibility. WBV has also been shown to help with disabling autoimmune and inflammatory conditions such as fibromyalgia and rheumatoid arthritis, and neurological conditions with mobility issues such as Parkinson's disease and multiple sclerosis. (See Chapter 4 for WBV's benefits for neurological conditions.)

One of the most obvious benefits of WBV for physical therapy is that it combines strength training without stressing the joints, since you don't have to move on the vibration plate to work muscles. By holding

WBV is effective therapy for a wide range of joint and movement issues.

different positions on the plate, you can target different muscles and joints (see Chapter 10 for illustrations). The intensity of the workout and stress on the joints can be adapted to varying levels of mobility, strength, and function.

Nothing convinces you not to move like pain, so WBV's powerful effects on pain levels are a critical part of mobility improvements. As discussed more thoroughly in Chapter 6, pain and inflammation levels often drop rapidly with WBV use. For the best results, especially for older people and autoimmune conditions such as rheumatic arthritis, it is important to use the right type of vibration machine and to start slowly and gently.

In my survey of my customers, using my machines and following my use guidelines, there was a reported drop in pain levels of 31 percent for many types (muscle, joint, back, and nerve) within weeks. While WBV does not work for everybody for pain reduction, it can be very dramatic for many, with 74 percent of those in pain reporting a 52 percent drop in their pain levels (see Appendix 1).

Flexibility also increases, especially when stretching positions are used, due to the automatic reflex response causing rapid involuntary tightening and relaxing of muscles. Muscle fibers will automatically tense and relax at the same rate as the vibration, twenty to eighty times per second, and the relaxation phase of this response rapidly and gently increases flexibility.

The automatic reflex response has a massage effect as well as a stretching effect that, along with relaxing tight muscles, increases circulation, bringing nutrients to the affected areas to aid in repair and regrowth. This massage effect happens automatically, but it can be heightened by placing the affected part of the body on the plate and relaxing. (One of my favorite positions for pure enjoyment and relaxation is a calf massage where you lie on your back, place your calves on the plate, cross your hands behind your head, and zone out.)

These stretching and massage effects can have rapid results. I have seen many people get on a machine and find that by the time they get off a few minutes later, painfully tight muscles have loosened, and they have a greater range of motion. Balance also improves because specialized nerve clusters that control balance (called proprioceptors) are stimulated, along with the rest of the nervous system. This is of particular benefit to the elderly who are at risk for dangerous falls.

Rheumatic Arthritis and Other Inflammatory Conditions

The ability of WBV to improve mobility is an important benefit for people with inflammatory and autoimmune conditions such as fibromyalgia and rheumatoid arthritis where mobility is decreased. Vibration improves mobility, which affects the health of other parts of the body such as bone, muscle, and other organs and systems.

WBV has also been shown to lower inflammation, as we saw earlier in this chapter, which might impact the progression of these diseases and damage to tissues from inflammation. More study is needed to determine the best regimens and conditions for success in these areas.[iii]

However, research on using WBV with inflammatory mobility conditions is encouraging. Previously we looked at a 2017 survey of the research on WBV and fibromyalgia. That study, while calling for more research on this subject due to small sample sizes and other study quality issues, did report significant improvements in fatigue and stiffness, along with decreasing pain levels for fibromyalgia sufferers.

> Several outcomes (based on the findings of one study) in this comparison [WBV versus control group] met the 15% threshold for clinical relevance: HRQL [health-relatedquality of life], pain intensity, fatigue, and stiffness, which improved by 16%, 39%, 46%, and 36%, respectively.[158]

Research on using WBV with rheumatoid arthritis has also shown improved mobility. A 2016 study of thirty-one women who had rheumatoid arthritis for at least three years found positive effects on

---

iii Note: Autoimmune conditions such as rheumatoid arthritis are listed under Relative Contraindications in Appendix 2. That means if WBV is used very carefully and possibly with additional support such as nutrition and supplements, this condition might improve with WBV (see Appendix 2: Contraindications).

functional ability and fatigue, as well as bone density.[159] In this study, half the women were randomly assigned to a control group where they continued with their normal activities, and the other half were given fifteen minutes of WBV twice a week for three months. The result was that functional ability and fatigue levels improved in the WBV group and either stayed the same or decreased in the control group. A further benefit was that while bone density decreased in the control group, there was no further loss of bone density in the WBV group. The article concluded, "Intermittent WBV shows promise for sustained improvements in functional ability, for attenuating loss of bone mass at the hip, as well as for decreasing fatigue in patients with established RA."[160]

For mobility problems due to nerve issues that are benefiting from the anti-inflammatory effects as well as intensely stimulated with vibration, there can be dramatic results. One of my clients, Richard Hawkins, a retired orthopedic surgeon, had been a lifelong runner before he lost his ability to run for seven years due to a mysterious peripheral nerve issue in his feet. I suspected mercury poisoning (he had been eating tuna fish every day for thirty years, and mercury is a potent neurotoxin) (see Chapter 8). I suggested some heavy metal detox products, a few homeopathics, diet changes, and vibration. From the very first session of vibration (one minute), he noticed an improvement, and within a few weeks of twice a week short sessions, he had begun to jog, with a big grin, to his car.

TESTIMONIAL

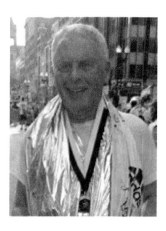

A lifelong runner, I gave up running at age sixty after developing numbness and pain in both feet. I spent seven years unable to run at all. I went to many different doctors, including specialists who told me there was nerve damage and that I would never get better, and I even tried surgery—all with no improvement. Then four years ago, I met Becky Chambers and started vibrating, increasing eventually to twenty minutes daily. I saw an improvement after the first session, and there has been a steady increase in function and feeling ever since. Now, four years later, I have just successfully completed this year's Boston Marathon, my twenty-seventh, at the age of seventy. Thanks, Becky Chambers!"

—Richard Hawkins, retired orthopedic surgeon

Vibrant Health's 2019 WBV Survey: Mobility

Using Vibrant Health machines, survey subjects reported an average 20–28 percent improvement in mobility, strength, and energy levels, along with an average 31 percent decrease in pain. Improvements often began within a few days.

In a 2019 survey of my company's Vibrant Health customers,[161] we asked respondents to rate their mobility before and after they began using WBV. Our survey subjects reported an average 20 to 28 percent improvement in mobility, strength, and energy levels, along with an average 31 percent decrease in pain within a few months of beginning their WBV program. Improvements often began within a few days. This survey is a testimony to my method. It is not meant to be a clinical trial but rather a guide for future research.

Chapter 8

Invigorating Your Immune System & Detoxing

In today's world of climate change and global interconnectedness and travel, our immune and detoxification systems are more important than ever. Weather extremes and other disasters are releasing unprecedented amounts of toxins into our environment and stressing our bodies. And the transmission of infectious viruses and other diseases can be breathtakingly rapid and potentially deadly. Keeping your health and immune system, including your lymphatic drainage and detoxification systems, in top working order is a must.

WBV invigorates and stimulates your body on every level. Ten minutes on the plate will feel like you have run a mile. Your blood zings through every blood vessel, your brain lights up, hormones increase, energy and mood rise—and all of them boost your immune system. WBV makes you feel alive—ten minutes, and your body will be tingling head to toe. It is common sense that WBV is good for your health, especially for people who are sedentary and getting very little stimulation.

The lymphatic system is a network of vessels, nodes, and organs that removes waste products and toxins from our body, and it is part of your immune system that protects you against infection and disease. This system relies on passive circulation. In other words, unlike blood vessels that require a heart to pump the blood around the body, there is no pump for the lymph system. The lymph system relies on your muscles tightening and relaxing around the lymph vessels to move the lymph, a process called lymph drainage. To keep this system working well, it is important to use your muscles regularly—another benefit of WBV.

WBV invigorates and stimulates your body on every level. Your blood zings through every blood vessel, your brain lights up, hormones increase, energy and mood rise—and all of them boost your immune system.

Your immune system is our defense against infections of all sorts, so keeping this circulation system working well is critical to your health and well-being. Some studies have shown a direct increase in immune-system, infection--fighting cells with WBV.[162,163] In addition, inflammation levels, which are mediated in part by your immune system, can decrease with WBV (see Chapter 2). This is indirect evidence that WBV is affecting your immune system in a positive way.

Many people think they should use powerful, high-amplitude vibration to get as much lymphatic drainage and movement as possible. *Do not do that.* Slow and steady is the best approach. Too much detoxing too quickly will make you worse. This problem is more common than many realize, especially when people who already have health problems use vibration machines.

Liberating toxins from where they are relatively safely stored in your body causes a sudden increase in work for your detox organs (primarily liver and kidneys), putting a strain on already overworked and stressed organs. That can lead to increased symptoms instead of relief. I have seen excessive detoxing innumerable times, including in myself.

You do not need high-amplitude vibration for lymphatic drainage and detoxing. Any vibration that travels throughout your entire body will be effective for this. In all my years of using vibration, I have *never* had a person *not* get enough detoxification, including clients with lymphedema (a sometimes painful swelling of arms or legs as lymph builds up in the tissues) and lipedema (an accumulation of excess fat in the legs)—two conditions for which improving lymphatic drainage is particularly important.

TESTIMONIALS

I got the Foot Vibrator for my mom when she woke up one day with lymphedema, in excruciating pain in her leg and couldn't walk. Using the foot vibrating machine twice a day was a large part of healing the lymphedema, and it didn't stop there. She now has more energy. It has helped relieve overall stress and brought relief to an old shoulder injury. My dad now uses it too. They're in their 80s.

—Kayde Witt

I have a disease in my legs called lipodema [a condition which can improve with increased lymphatic drainage]. There is no cure, and it is extremely painful. I've had it for many years, but it got really bad since menopause. All the time, I felt like I had lumps of lead in my legs and they were aching all the time. Walking became impossible, other than very slowly for short distances.

I've been doing WBV for one and a half years along with energy medicine counseling with Becky Chambers, and the pain is now 80–90 percent better. I have not taken any painkiller meds in the last two months! I could not live without my WBV. I could tell that the WBV was helping me because within a few weeks of starting it, I began to feel a certain lightness in my legs that I had not felt in years and years.

I have gone to gyms and all kinds of exercise places. I tell them all about my issue, and they would give me exercises. Strengthening muscles is important, but it is the increased flow of lymph that really helps me. WBV is everything all at once. It has been a lifesaver for me.

—Urvashi B.

Wow! After using my new foot vibration shaker for the first time for only 10 minutes, I was in for a great surprise! I had my feet on it early in the evening before my last two clients and had been standing, working on clients all day, then sitting at my desk doing paperwork for several hours. When I took my socks off last night, there was no swelling. I normally have some level of edema and very impaired circulation in my legs—varicose veins since my late teens and tons of scar tissue from vein stripping and ablations, so some level of swelling is pretty much a given even with all I do to keep blood and lymph moving.

I noticed improved mobility in my feet and ankles after two days and no leg cramps during the night since I've been using it this last week. I like the lowest speed with the shiatsu massage and the second and third speed without it for more intense vibration. It is very quiet, too, which was really important to me. I'm excited to share this wellness tool with my clients who have desk jobs or stand at work all day. What a quick and easy way to improve blood and lymphatic flow!

—Dawn O., wellness spa owner

Toxins Everywhere

Our environment is loaded with toxins, and despite our best attempts to avoid them, some of these toxins end up in our bodies. In a PBS television special several years ago, Bill Moyers, a typical healthy person, had his blood tested at Mt. Sinai School of Medicine. Eighty-four different and highly toxic chemicals were found in his body.[164]

Once in our bodies, toxins may cause damage and disease. Toxins have been linked to almost all chronic health issues. Sherry A. Rogers, MD, a leading authority on environmental medicine, writes this in her 2002 book *Detoxify or Die:*

Pesticides, volatile organic hydrocarbons, auto and industrial pollution, mycotoxins, heavy metals, and more mimic any disease. They can cause any symptom or disease from high blood pressure, heart failure, osteoporosis, high cholesterol, arthritis, or Alzheimer's disease to fibromyalgia, degenerating disks, Parkinson's disease, depression, fatigue, irritable bowel, loss of libido, colitis, asthma, eczema, prostatitis, esophagitis, atrial fibrillation, GERD (gastroesophageal reflux disease), hearing loss, headaches, recurrent sinus, ear or throat infections, diabetes or cancer, and more.[165]

TESTIMONIAL

I'm impressed with the speed in which I noticed shifts in my energy and mood. Taylor Swift's song "Shake It Off" came to mind daily to remind me to let go of the old and vibrate into the new. I'm an ND (naturopathic doctor). I was in good health when I started and was more curious about improving strength. Nonetheless I am glad that I listened to the advice to start slowly because I did have some detox symptoms show up early on, which wasn't really a surprise because I had been ignoring some symptoms for some time. But soon enough, I was up to 10–20 minutes a day, detoxing easily and feeling overall more vital and optimistic about life. I will stand, dance, or do resistance training on my vibration plate. I am so very grateful for all the work and research that Becky Chambers put into crafting this machine and taking care and consideration of the nervous system harmonization. I am so glad I bought the Power 1000 and have recommended it to friends and clients.

—Dr. Joylyn Sparkles

What Should One Do?

A regular detoxification program is a wise idea for everybody, and it is essential for people with chronic health issues. Remember, however, that detoxification should be done with caution since detoxing is stressful for the body and can cause an increase in symptoms for someone with an already weakened body. Your body has natural systems to eliminate and neutralize toxins through the colon, liver, kidneys, lymphatic system, lungs, and skin. However, with the buildup of toxicity levels in your body and the consequent breakdown of health, it is important to support and aid your body in this process.

A key benefit of vibration is that it is a powerful aid to your natural detoxification process. When vibrating, all your muscle fibers involuntarily tense and relax at the same rate the machine is vibrating, twenty to eighty times per second. This creates a powerful massage for your lymphatic system, which is one of the body's primary natural detoxing tools.

The muscle workout provided by WBV leads to an increased flow of the lymph moving toxins out of your body; [also the] increased circulation brings more nutrients and oxygen to all the cells.

Unlike the heart and blood, this system does not have its own pumping system. Muscles contracting around lymphatic vessels force the lymph (a clear fluid) to move. The muscle workout provided by WBV thus leads to an increased flow of the lymph, moving toxins out of your body. In addition, increased circulation brings more nutrients and oxygen to all the cells, helping them function at a higher level and therefore dumping more toxins and waste products into the lymph.

The position you hold on the plate determines which muscles are activated, so I advise using a variety of positions. Standing upright on the plate will activate the muscles in your lower body and torso but not your arms. To increases lymphatic drainage in your arms, do some exercise positions where your hands are on the plate (such as push-ups) or arm massages where you rest your arms on the plate.

Detox Overload

Detoxing with WBV is so powerful that it is the major limiting factor for most people using WBV, not muscle strength as many people assume. Detoxing will happen anytime you are on a machine, whether you just stand there or are actively exercising. As with detoxing after a massage or sauna or any other detox system, it is possible to overload your already stressed detox pathways and have a temporary increase in symptoms.

Common detox symptoms are exhaustion, headaches, and digestive problems, but any health issue that is linked to toxins can temporarily worsen as more toxins are released into the circulatory system. In fact, since any health problem you already have is a "weak link" in your system, when you overstress your body with detoxing, that weak link is a likely place to show the strain.

Candida yeast problems are also likely to flare up with detox overload. Since the liver is your major detox organ and is also part of the immune system, under the increased strain, your immune system may be overloaded with work, and this opportunistic parasite is likely to flare up. In fact, a *Candida* yeast flare-up is a likely sign that you are in detox overload and need to do less vibration and possibly take a detox support supplement. Detox reactions are an enlightening opportunity to see the close connection between toxins and chronic health issues, something that is not always recognized by Western medicine.

Detox problems often do not show up until six to twenty-four hours after using WBV. So even though the vibration feels gentle and pleasant, use caution! Start slowly, and increase slowly. Many people do best starting with just one minute on a gentle, low-power machine (see Chapter 9).

> *Detox problems often do not show up until six to twenty-four hours after using WBV. So . . . use caution!*

What to Do If You Experience Detox Overload

If any existing symptoms worsen or new ones suddenly appear, it is possible that toxins are involved. You should stop vibrating and rest a few days. If symptoms decrease, you can start up again with less vibration. You can aid your body with detoxing by drinking extra water and juice to help flush out toxins and by getting plenty of sleep. Additionally, the over-the-counter products below are designed to remove toxins. Follow the directions on the package, and always check with your doctor or medical professional before starting something new.

- ♦ **Activated charcoal:** This product very effectively absorbs toxins, but be sure to take this product on an empty stomach (one hour before food or two hours after food) because it will absorb nutrients as well as toxins.

- ♦ **Modified citrus pectin:** This is a great product (sold under several different brand names; I usually use PectaSol) that will be absorbed into your bloodstream, go everywhere in your body, and absorb only toxins. It can be taken with or without food.

- ♦ **UltraClear Plus:** This liver-support nutritional powder provides enhanced support for balanced metabolic detoxification, including macro- and micronutrients to address liver function. The formula includes glycine and L-cysteine to help support Phase II liver detoxification. Green tea catechins and beta-carotene provide protection against potentially harmful compounds generated during the natural liver detoxification process. It is also high in antioxidants (beta-carotene and vitamins C and E) to provide additional nutritional support.

Consult a natural healthcare practitioner for your specific situation. Sometimes additional products or homeopathics are needed to resolve a situation.

Chapter 9

Different Types of Whole Body Vibration Machines

Over the last twenty-five years, I have used and sold many different vibration machines. My personal experience with my own health and the results I have seen with hundreds of my clients have shown me that the type of machine you use, especially with seniors and others with health challenges, can be important to the success of whole body vibration.

Since I had problems using a double motor machine (see Chapter 4), I am careful about which whole body vibration machines I use and recommend. Eventually, using my knowledge and experience, I designed and developed my own machines to ensure that I have a reliable supply of the kind of machines I recommend for my clients and customers.

With the increasing popularity of whole body vibration, there has been a surge of interest in making and selling vibration machines, resulting in a plethora of confusing promotional information. Some manufacturers claim their machines are "vertical motion" when they are not. Some claim their machines are high-frequency vibration when they are not. I can only recommend with complete confidence my own machines and others you will find on my website.

For your convenience, my machines are listed below. If you want to understand the field and options for other types of machines, more information follows, but be prepared. It can be an overwhelming jungle of information. My machines are available on my website, and some of them are also available on Amazon. Check my website (www. BCVibrantHealth.com) for the latest information.

The most important information for many people is that you don't need to spend a great deal of money to get enormous benefit. There is a huge range of machines, and you can get an effective and therapeutic device for less than an annual gym membership and much less than what you might spend on healthcare. Considering all the benefits to your health, you will likely end up saving a great deal of money.

Currently, there are three Vibrant Health machines: two vibration platforms and a small foot vibration device. My machines are designed to heal, but exactly what goes into creating this vibration is complicated. I list the amplitude of my machines, along with other information, because it is important, but do not decide on a machine based solely on those specifications. For more information, you can read the information later in this chapter on g-force, amplitude, and frequency. There are many factors that go into creating vibration. My machines are based on years of trying many machines and studying the effects, particularly for people with chronic health issues. My results—which you can see in Appendix 1, on my website, and

I believe that the clarity of the electromagnetic signal from a single motor, vertical vibration machine contributes to the results I achieve.

in my books—are your assurance that my machines will provide you with what you need.

I believe that the clarity of the electromagnetic signal from a single motor, vertical vibration machine contributes to the results I achieve. There are also many other excellent machines out there, and I suggest that you consult with your health practitioner who knows your health needs.

1. VIBRANT HEALTH POWER 1000: As Vibrant Health's most popular model, this machine delivers a vibration powerful enough to give you an intense workout, but it is still gentle enough to be safe and easy to use. It is designed for people of all ages. It is especially ideal for children, busy adults, Baby Boomers, and older. *(If you are very fragile with age or illness, please see below for low intensity vibration (LIV) using the Ultimate Vibe machine).* The Vibrant Health Power 1000 is the perfect machine for optimizing both physical and mental health with a carefully designed, perfectly synchronized, smooth vibration. It delivers a challenging workout or deep massage and a stretch for tight muscles. It is the best vibration for brain function and brain wave synchronization. Standing upright on this plate, you will feel the vibration travel through your entire body and up into your head—but don't worry, it feels good and is not bad for you.

The vertical vibration motion of this machine feels like a powerful cheetah purring (though probably not as quietly). Because this motion is smooth, the average person with normal balance will not need a handle to hold onto. If you do have balance issues, you can buy an optional tower and handle to go with the machine, use a separate balance bar, or put the vibration plate next to something to hold on to. There are also two kinds of straps—stretchy and non-stretchy—for use with different arm exercise positions.

Frequency range: 26–45 Hz

Motor Amplitude*: 1.5–3.0 mm*

Plate Amplitude* (Hi): 1.0–1.5 mm*

Cost: $995

Available through www.BCVibrantHealth.com and
authorized distributors.

*These are the highest amplitudes for high-frequency, vertical vibration machines that I recommend for your total health and well-being. Plate amplitude is different from motor amplitude (some companies only report motor amplitude). A vibration that is too strong can harm your musculature and neurological systems, which can negatively impact your entire body. (More information about maximum safe amplitudes and gravitational forces can be found later in this chapter.) Amplitude measurements reported here are peak to peak. Lower amplitude value is with a 160-pound person on the machine; higher value is with no additional weight on the vibration platform.

2. VIBRANT HEALTH ULTIMATE VIBE: Twenty plus years of research and building ever-better vibration machines have resulted in the creation of the new Ultimate Vibe machine. It is designed to work for all conditions and goals for which you might want to use whole body vibration, as described in my whole body vibration books. From athletic performance to immune system boosting, from increasing bone density to losing weight, from lowering inflammation to dealing with more severe chronic health conditions, the Ultimate Vibe will give you what you need.

Whether you are new to vibration, fragile, older, dealing with significant health issues, or are a healthy and athletic younger person looking to take your level of athletic performance, endurance, and health to another level, this machine will work for you. The Ultimate Vibe machine is a breakthrough in vibration technology, combining in one machine both low and high power settings and a wide range of frequencies (15–40 Hz).

The low power setting delivers low intensity vibration (LIV). This extremely gentle vibration with a very low amplitude (0.1 mm) and g-force (0.3–0.4g) is safe for almost any situation and person (see more about low intensity vibration (LIV) later in this chapter).

The high power setting delivers the maximum safe amplitude. (More information about maximum safe amplitudes and gravitational forces can be found later in this chapter.) The intensity on the high (and low) power settings can be modified further from gentler to stronger by the wide range of frequency settings (15–40 Hz) that are available.

The result is a machine that can produce vibration with the extreme gentleness necessary for debilitating and severe chronic health issues and the greater force and power needed for an athletic, intense workout with its more effective weight loss and bone, muscle, and joint strengthening. Many people with less severe chronic conditions may also benefit from starting with the very gentle low power setting and graduating to the high power setting as their health improves.

An optional handle is available and can be added to the machine at any time. However, if your balance is normal, you will likely not need a handle since the vibration is very smooth.

Frequency range: 15–40 Hz

Two Power/Amplitude settings:

Low Power: low intensity vibration (LIV)

Motor Amplitude*: 0.7–1.2 mm*

Plate Amplitude* 0.1–0.5 mm*

High Power:

Motor Amplitude*: 1.5–3.0 mm*

Plate Amplitude* (Hi): 1.0–1.5 mm*

Optional Handle

Cost: $599

Available on: www.BCVibrantHealth.com

or Amazon: Search for "BC Vibrant Health Ultimate
   Vibe Vibration Plate Exercise Machine"

or use this link:

  https://www.amazon.com/dp/B07D3BZRS8

*The high power setting has the highest amplitude for high frequency vertical vibration machines that I recommend for your total health and well-being. Plate amplitude is different from motor amplitude. A vibration that is too strong can harm your musculature and neurological systems, which can negatively impact your entire body. (More information about maximum safe amplitudes and gravitational forces can be found later in this chapter.) Amplitude measurements reported here are peak to peak. Lower amplitude value is with a 160-pound person on the machine; a higher value is with no additional weight on the vibration platform.

3. VIBRANT HEALTH FOOT VIBRATING MASSAGE SHAKER: Foot vibration machines are a new option for people who are fragile and older or not yet ready to invest in a bigger, more expensive machine but still want to dip their feet into vibration technology. These devices are lightweight, small, inexpensive, and easy—you just sit on a chair next to the device and put your feet on it or lie on the ground and rest your legs on it. Since they are smaller and lighter weight, you can also take them with you when you travel.

Automatic foot and leg movements trigger muscle fibers to tighten and relax nerves, shooting signals to your brain to wake it up. Circulation increases, bringing nutrients and oxygen to your tissues and removing waste products. The machine is also good for lymphatic drainage and detoxification as your leg and foot muscle fibers massage and move toxins through your lymphatic system. In theory, as with other forms of vibration, the stimulation of your nervous system, brain, and body may lead to lower stress levels and thus inflammation levels, though less powerfully than other more powerful vibration machines.

The direction of motion is vertical, but it is a different system that allows the heels of your feet to move more than your toes, causing a shaking motion that gives your leg muscles exercise. Since you cannot stand or put much weight on these devices, the more intensive, full body exercise options that are available with larger vibration machines are not possible.

Other companies also offer foot vibrating devices. Be careful not to get a device that only delivers massage or electrical stimulation and not vibration. They feel good but won't deliver the same benefits.

Note that some of my fragile clients start on this foot massage machine and then as they become stronger, opt for a standing vibration machine.

3 vibration speeds plus massage

Cost: $149

Available through www.BCVibrantHealth.com

Double Motor Vibration Machines

As discussed earlier, many whole body vibration (WBV) machines have two motors in them. These machines provide greater power, but I feel they are not appropriate for anyone other than the very strong, athletic Olympic-level or professional athletes that these machines were originally designed for. To get in top shape or to heal illness, your body and mind will need a different approach.

Two motors can also send an asynchronized signal into the nervous system (see "My Experience with Desynchronization" in Chapter 4), which theoretically could have deleterious effects on the brain and nervous system. My reason for not recommending these machines is twofold: first, my personal experience with this type of machine when I suddenly developed problems that resolved only when I switched to a single motor, fully synchronized machine; and second, my success with coaching others who are dealing with health issues or are older. These two factors have led me to recommend and use only single motor, fully synchronized machines. There is more to vibration than just getting the workout. There is the impact on your whole body and brain to consider, and you can still get a great workout with a single motor machine.

Different Models and Makes

There are many companies now selling vibration machines, and some machines are sold by different distributors under different names, sometimes for widely varying prices, which makes it hard to know exactly what type of vibration they are offering. I will try to clarify, but because this is a booming field with many companies using different terms, often for the same thing, it is difficult to discern the differences. That is why I recommend my own machines so I know exactly what you are getting and what I believe will safely give you the desired results.

Vibration machines were first developed (and are still best known) for their ability to create an intense workout. Many WBV machine companies have the football-player mindset that the more power the better. Thus, many of the best-selling machines and most of the machines you will find in health clubs and sports centers are the double motor variety of vertical motion machines. They produce a large amplitude and g-force with a different type of motion called "oscillation" (see explanation below). Beyond this issue, there are several other variables to consider: direction of movement, power (g-force), amplitudes, frequencies, durability, and cost.

Direction of Movement

Vertical (Linear) Motion vs. Oscillation Motion

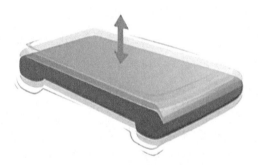

Vertical Motion

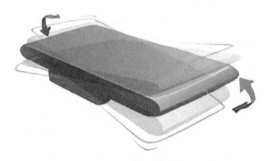

Oscillation

VERTICAL VIBRATION MOTION

There are two major types of motion for vibration plates. Vertical, or linear, motion machines vibrate mostly up and down. This is the type of machine I recommend for most people. Some companies have renamed other motions with this vertical vibration. For example, I have seen a very different motion called oscillation motion (see image on the previous page and discussion below) labeled "vertical vibration," which can be quite confusing.

When the vertical vibration is a true vertical up and down motion, it provides a smooth wave of vibration through your body, your nervous system, and your brain. If this motion is too strong (as can happen with high g-force and amplitude machines), the vibration can be stressful for your body. Therefore, I only recommend vibration machines with gentle to moderate levels of vertical vibration that will not stress your body.

There is also a wide variety of terms used to describe slight variations on vertical vibration such as three-dimensional, horizontal, spiral, circular, tri-planar, triangular, tri-phasic, multidimensional, omniflex, and piston. These terms are often describing double motor machine motions that are basically the same type of vertical motion with an additional very slight horizontal or circular motion. Because there can be an asynchronous vibration created from double motor machines, I do not recommend this type of machine for most people.

WBV machines also vary widely in amplitudes, g-force, durability, and cost. The intensity of your vibration workout depends on the power, or gravitational force (g-force), of the vibration—a factor that takes into account the amplitude and frequency of the vibration and the weight (your own weight) that your muscles must hold against the vibration. Since amplitudes, frequency, and your weight can vary greatly, the intensity of your workout can also vary.

It helps to understand the terms. Vibration machines vary in type of motion: vertical (up and down) or oscillating (a seesaw type motion). They also vary in amplitude, g-force, and frequency. In buying a machine, get to know the terms below.

Amplitude: A measure of how far the plate moves up and down during each unit of movement.

G-Force (sometimes referred to as intensity): To get a sense of what g-force means, imagine putting your hand on a purring cat versus holding onto a jackhammer. These are very different experiences due to the different amplitudes and weights involved. A jackhammer's amplitude of vibration and its weight are much greater than the weight of the cat and its amplitude of motion when purring. So even though the frequencies of these vibrations are similar, the total g-force, and therefore effect, is greater for the jackhammer.

Frequency: The rate at which something occurs or is repeated over a particular period of time. In the case of vibration plates, frequency refers to the number of times the plate moves up and down in one second. Vibrations per second are expressed as "Hz."

Frequency ranges for vertical vibration machines are typically 20–50 Hz. The range includes bone and muscle development optimal frequencies of 30–35 Hz and higher frequencies that may be particularly helpful for the brain and nervous system.

OSCILLATION VIBRATION MOTION

Oscillation motion is like having one foot on either end of a seesaw, with one foot rising while the other one is falling, back and forth. People on an oscillating vibration machine will be moving very noticeably. In contrast, when a person is using a vertical vibration machine, you cannot see them vibrating. Oscillation vibration is also sometimes called pivotal, or teeter-totter. Some companies call this oscillating motion "vertical vibration," which is confusing.

These machines can provide a wide range of amplitudes and g-forces since the amplitude can be adjusted by the position of your feet on the plate, and they usually have adjustable speeds. You can get a good workout with high g-forces or a gentle walking type effect. Oscillation vibration machines generally have higher maximum amplitudes and lower frequencies than vertical vibration machines. One reason that oscillation vibration machines generally run slower may be due to the greater motion (than with vertical vibration) that is created in your body as one foot rises while the other falls. If the speed is high at the same time as the amplitude of motion, this movement might be too fast for comfort. Oscillation machines usually have a range of frequencies from 1–20 Hz, although some companies make machines that go up to 30–35 Hz. The actual frequency of vibration can sometimes be hard to discern since some oscillation machines have an arbitrary speed scale that might be, for example, 1–100, but there is not a unit designation so you don't know the vibrations per second (Hz).

Many people report great results with this type of machine, and there is a lot of research on these machines. They can create an excellent workout, and they are particularly effective for increasing circulation and lymphatic drainage. The larger movements created by oscillation motion can also sometimes be great for loosening stiff joints and muscles.

HYBRID-MOTION MACHINES

There are now machines that have multiple types of motion controlled by multiple motors within one device. They can have up to three motors in them with three different types of motion—the two described above and a motion they label "horizontal." They also often have the option of operating multiple motions at one time, which I would not recommend. These machines have not been studied much yet.

Typically, these machines give you a little bit of everything but not enough of the type of vibration I prefer—true vertical vibration.

SONIC VIBRATION

The final type of machine has a true vertical (linear) vibration motion that is generated by sonic (sound) waves. No actual sound is produced by these machines; the term "sonic" is used to describe a sound wave type of mechanism that produces a vertical movement, not a sound. These machines typically create smooth, synchronized vibrations with a large range of amplitudes as well as frequencies, but the cost is also very high ($3,000 to $10,000) without significant additional benefits for the average user.

Remember, a greater amplitude and g-force do not mean better results! The machines I most often recommend are $600 to $1,000.

Intense exercise is only one of many benefits you can get from vibration. For many people, if they try to work out too intensely with vibration at the beginning, they will end up feeling worse instead of better because of too much stress on the body and nervous system, and too much detoxing. Be patient! Remember, you can get exercise many ways. The workout effect is not the only benefit, and it is not what makes vibration so unique. Muscle strength, toning, and weight loss are only the tip of the iceberg when it comes to vibration's benefits.

Gravitational (g) Force, Amplitude, and Frequency

The power of a machine (g-force) is determined by the amplitude (the distance the plate moves), the frequency (the rate or speed of vibration), and the weight of the person on the plate.[iv] The greater the amplitude, the frequency, and the weight, the greater the g-force. Again, imagine putting your hand on a purring cat versus holding a jackhammer—these are very different experiences because of the different amplitudes and weights involved, even though the frequencies of vibration are similar. G-force is a common way people compare machines, although it is not an exact method since people's weights vary significantly, and weight is a component for determining g-force.

Changing the amplitude dramatically changes the g-force. Until recently, to change the amplitude of a single motor vertical vibration machine, you usually needed to change machines.

Recent advances in vibration technology have led to the creation of machines with only one motor that are able to change the amplitude of vibration—a critical determinant of the g-force of a vibration machine—with the press of a button (see the Ultimate Vibe at the beginning of this chapter). This is an important breakthrough since people with more health issues sometimes need to start with a very gentle vibration and later, as their health improves, switch to a higher amplitude vibration.

FAQ: What is the maximum amplitude and g-force I should use when vibrating?

G-force and amplitude have become a hot topic, with many consumers searching for high numbers. This market pressure has led to inflating g-force and amplitude numbers. It is like women's dress sizes—we get bigger, but dress sizes stay the same or go down . . . because

---

iv   This assumes the *plate* amplitude is used for g-force calculations, as this will automatically account for the weight of the plate.

that is how we want to think!

G-force (or intensity of vibration) is calculated by a complicated mathematical equation that includes the amplitude and frequency of the machine and the weight of the person. Further complicating such determinations of g-force is the condition that as the weight on the machine increases, the amplitude will generally decrease due to the increased workload on the motor to move that weight.

The short answer to the question of maximum amplitude is that for total health and safety—*when using the single motor, high frequency, vertical vibration type of machine I recommend*[v]—you should use nothing above a plate amplitude of 2.0 mm (peak to peak movement).[vi] A vibration that is too strong can harm your musculature and neurological systems. Note that there is a

To be totally safe, my machines have a maximum plate amplitude of 1.5 millimeters. This amount of vibration will give you a good workout and bone density signal. Maximum recommended length of time vibrating under these conditions is 10–20 minutes per day. As emphasized in all my books, anyone new to vibration should start slowly, with the low amplitude and frequency settings, and gradually work up to the higher settings.

---

v   This recommendation is for vertical vibration machines only. Since oscillation machines run more slowly, they create lower g-forces at equivalent amplitudes, so higher amplitudes can be used.

vi In response to people wanting high-amplitude (high-power) machines and making buying decisions based on this factor, many companies now use a peak-to-peak measurement of amplitude versus a more traditional centerline-to-peak amplitude measurement. Using the peak-to-peak measurement method produces amplitudes twice as big as the centerline method without actually changing the true vibration. Other companies deal with this issue by not giving amplitude information at all. When amplitude information is given, there is generally no explanation or consensus for which measurement is being referenced.

difference between motor amplitude and plate amplitude. Plate amplitude is what you actually feel and receive when you are standing on the machine. Motor amplitude is the amount of movement from the motor alone. Some companies report only the motor amplitude.

To be totally safe, my machines have a maximum plate amplitude of 1.5 millimeters, resulting in a maximum g-force for users of approximately 1.0 g during workouts. This amount of vibration will give you a good workout and bone density signal. Maximum recommended length of time vibrating under these conditions is 10–20 minutes per day. As emphasized in all my books, anyone new to vibration should start slowly with the low amplitude and frequency settings, and gradually work up to the higher settings.

Double motor, vertical, or linear-motion machines can deliver high amplitudes along with high frequencies and thus g-forces, but as noted earlier, I don't recommend these machines. Oscillating motion machines also often have high maximum amplitudes, but when the frequency is low, as is often the case for these machines, the g-force will also be lower.

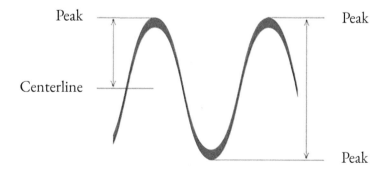

LOW INTENSITY VIBRATION (LIV)

Low intensity vibration, or LIV, is an extremely gentle and safe type of vibration. For elderly and more fragile people worried about bone density, this high speed, very low amplitude (< 0.5 mm) vertical vibration can be the best choice because of its extreme gentleness and safety. These machines generate very low gravitational forces (0.3–0.4 g), which is less impact than generated by walking across the living room floor, in a vertical vibration motion. While it is not as powerful and effective for bone and muscle as a higher amplitude vibration, there are very few contraindications. LIV is excellent for more fragile people such as the elderly and those struggling with more severe health challenges, and it can be a steppingstone to using a stronger type of vibration.

Vibrant Health's Ultimate Vibe machines are designed to provide the benefits of the extremely gentle LIV workout but with the capacity to move up the stronger g-force and amplitude that is more effective for bone density and workout effects.

WHAT IS THE BEST FREQUENCY TO USE?

Much effort has gone into figuring out which frequencies, types of motion, and positions on the machine are best for losing weight and cellulite, increasing bone density and muscle strength, lymph drainage, and so on. My experience is that focusing on exactly what frequency is best for achieving certain effects is usually a moot point. By far the most important issue is to start at a low frequency and increase slowly so you lower inflammation and stress, allowing your body and mind to heal itself.

However, as you become able to tolerate the higher frequencies, the question of what frequency is best for a particular issue becomes more important, and higher settings can be beneficial and do have more powerful effects. *Always go slowly,* or you may end up disappointed and stop entirely. But on the other hand, as long as you are using my machines and following my guidelines for using them, you will be safe and can gradually work up to using the higher amplitude and frequency settings.

See the "Optimal Frequency Settings" section in the next chapter for recommendations on specific frequencies for different purposes. Also see my book *Whole Body Vibration for Seniors* for physical therapy guidelines and recommendations for specific health issues.

Remember that even gentle vibration will affect your whole body and give you anti-inflammatory effects. So no matter what frequency or amplitude of a single motor, vertical vibration machine you use, as long as you also do not do too much and overstress your body, you will be on your way to lowering inflammation and achieving the desired results.

Durability

Durability depends on the machine's quality of construction. Plastic parts are not as durable as steel, but for low-cost, low–g-force machines, plastic can be a reasonable option. Larger, more powerful machines are usually made of metal and can weigh quite a lot. Many machines are made overseas and shipped to the United States. Quality can vary widely, so be sure to check the warranty terms and weight limits for users. Generally, the higher the g-force and amplitude of a machine, the larger, heavier, and more expensive it will likely be. That is because the motor must be more powerful to generate greater amplitude, and since vibration tends to shake things apart, the machine must be built to withstand increasing force.

Cost

There is an enormous range in the cost of machines. You can spend $150 for a small foot vibration device or $200 for an inexpensive oscillation machine, but up to $13,000 for some sonic vibration machines and everything in between. The cost depends on many factors, including the type of machine and amount of power, the quality of construction, the availability of knowledgeable customer support, as well as demand and marketing strategy.

Remember, you don't need to spend a huge amount of money to get an excellent machine and experience the benefits of WBV!

Chapter 10

Getting Started with Whole Body Vibration

In this chapter are daily plans for how to get started, a beginner's program, and guidelines for more advanced users. Whole body vibration is an intensive workout,

The sooner you start your natural health regimen, the better!

but for most people, it won't make you sweat or feel exhausted—so jump right in!

First, be sure to check the contraindications listed in Appendix 2. Also, before starting any therapeutic and/or exercise program, it is advisable to discuss WBV therapy with your physician.

There is a huge variation in how people respond to vibration. If you do not have any health problems and you are feeling great with WBV, you can increase your time and speed at a much faster pace. A healthy young person might be able to do ten minutes on a powerful machine and feel fine the first time they use it. Other people, especially those with health issues, may need months just to get to ten minutes at the lowest speed on a low-power machine.

For example, I had a sixty-year-old client with chronic fatigue and depression who experienced a dramatic improvement in energy and mood after his first one-minute session at the lowest frequency on a gentle machine. He did not have a long history of health issues, though, and had a robust constitution. He was able to increase to ten minutes at the highest frequency within a couple of months.

At the other end of the spectrum is me. I have a long history of health problems and am a very sensitive person, so it took me years to get to the highest setting on the same gentle machine while also taking an impressive number of nutritional products and using other types of natural health therapies.

For improving the general health and well-being for people with chronic health issues, the goal is to gradually increase the length of the daily vibration session to at least ten minutes at a frequency of 30 Hz on a single motor vertical vibration machine.

> *Note: Ideally you are using the stronger, higher power/amplitude level of vibration I recommend (which I have referred to at times as mid-level amplitude or sometimes even "relatively gentle" to distinguish it from the very high power/amplitude double motor machines that I do not recommend). But if necessary, you can use extremely low intensity vibration (LIV) (see Chapter 8 for details on machines).*

This amount of WBV supplies many benefits every day. If you are having problems of any sort, stop vibrating altogether, and see if you get better. If you do, try less vibration. Keep in mind that any vibration can have dramatic positive effects, so start slowly. Increase at your own pace—and enjoy!

Whole Body Vibration Training Basics

Goals

♦ *Minimum recommended usage (but work up to this slowly):* 10 minutes of vibration each day at a frequency setting of 30–35 Hz at a mid-level power/amplitude setting (the Power 1000 machine or high power setting on the Ultimate Vibe). It is not a problem if you miss some days. It is great if you can work up to doing 20 minutes per day.

If you are using the extremely gentle LIV type of machine, you should aim for 10 minutes twice a day with at least 5–6 hours between sessions.

♦ *Maximum recommended usage:* 20 minutes of vibration per day for the more powerful type of machine I recommend, such as the Vibrant Health Power 1000. LIV machines (such as the Ultimate Vibe on low power) and foot vibe devices are so gentle that you can do 40 minutes per day.

Basics

♦ To target different muscle groups, choose different positions from the pictures in this book or from the poster found on my website.

♦ If you have a foot vibration device, follow the recommendations in the beginner's program for increasing time and speed. Depending on your health, you may be able to increase more rapidly since the effect is smaller. This device is mostly used by sitting in a chair next to it and putting your feet on it. You cannot stand or sit on the machine. You can, however, massage your legs and get vibration higher up in your legs by lying on the floor with your calves or thighs resting on the foot pads of the device.

♦ Do each exercise position for 30 seconds to 1 minute, either holding the position (static, or isometric) or moving in and out of it (dynamic, or kinetic).

♦ Many benefits are achieved even if you only stand on the machine. In fact, standing upright on the plate is a great position for increasing bone density since it helps transmit the vibration throughout your body. Even if you are too tired to work out, do stand or sit on your plate—relax and vibrate!

♦ **Optimal Frequency Settings**
    Low frequencies (15–30 Hz) are perfect for warm-ups, cool-downs, getting started with WBV, and slowly building up your health and tolerance.
    Mid-level frequencies (30–35 Hz) are optimal for muscle and bone strengthening, exercise, stretching, and massage. Some research indicates that 30 Hz may be ideal for bone and muscle growth.
    High frequencies (35–50 Hz) are ideal for the brain and nervous system.

In the beginning, don't worry about using an optimal speed for working out or another purpose. *The most important thing is to start slowly and just do some vibration!* Remember that *all* vibration on the right kind of machine—and not too much that can overstress your body—will help lower inflammation and achieve strengthening, stretching, massage, lymphatic drainage, and other health benefits.

Becky Chambers'
Slow and Gentle Beginner's Program

These guidelines have been developed particularly with my machines in mind. I cannot vouch for their applicability to other types of machines.

DAY 1: Stand on your vibration machine for a short amount of time (30 seconds to 5 minutes, depending on which machine you are using; see below*) at **the lowest frequency/speed setting**.

WBV has very powerful effects on every part of your body, so I recommend starting with a very small amount of vibration on the first day to see how you respond. Watch and wait for 24 hours before trying any more vibration. As long as you feel the same or better the next day, you can increase the length of time of your next vibration session.

Increasing the frequency is a big step up; so first increase the length of time you are on the machine, getting up to 10 minutes at the same frequency setting before increasing the frequency (speed) setting by one increment.

Some people will be able to increase the amount of WBV much faster than other people. If you find that you are feeling better and having no problems following the beginner's program, then you can try increasing your time and speed more rapidly.

Relatively Gentle machine: start with 30–60 seconds

LIV machines or Foot Vibe: start with 5 minutes

DAY 2: Increase the time by a small amount,* staying at the same low speed. More sensitive people should do the same amount of time for 2–5 days before increasing.

Relatively Gentle machine: 30–60 seconds

LIV machines: 5 minutes

Foot Vibe devices have fewer speed settings, so stay at the same time longer before increasing the speed.

EACH FOLLOWING DAY (or every 2–5 days): Increase the time incrementally** without increasing the speed. Go up to a total of 10 minutes for Relatively Gentle vibration, or 20 minutes for LIV.

- When you get to the desired session length, drop the time down to 3–5 minutes, but increase the speed one setting. Increase the time again at this new speed following the same guidelines as above.

- As you gradually increase the speed, one setting at a time, continue to follow this same pattern of increasing the amount of time day by day, and dropping the time back down when you increase the speed setting.

Relatively Gentle machine: 30–60 seconds
LIV machines or Foot Vibe: 5 minutes

FAQS

Q. Can I use my vibration machine more than once a day?
A. Yes, but the total amount of time per day needs to stay the same. In other words, if you have been slowly building up and are now doing 10 minutes per day without any problems, you can split that into a 5-minute morning session and a 5-minute evening session. You cannot suddenly start doing 10 minutes morning and night without risking overdosing on your vibration.

Q. Does it matter what time of the day I use my machine?
A. Many people love to use the vibration in the morning to wake themselves up and set themselves up for a great day. Others might want to split up their time during the day for quick rejuvenating breaks. Some people find that an evening session is just the ticket for relaxing and helping them sleep. Any of these approaches are fine. However, some people find that vibrating in the evening is too stimulating for them, and they have trouble falling asleep afterward. So if you try that and it doesn't work for you, no harm done. Just do your vibration earlier in the day.

Q. Why does my nose (ear, feet, or any other body part) itch while I am vibrating?
A. We don't really know, but there are theories. One theory is that

an increase in blood coming to the surface of the skin due to an increase in circulation causes itchiness. Other theories are that the itchiness could be a type of detoxing or energetic effect. The good news is that as long as the itching is temporary and goes away shortly after you stop vibrating, it is just a temporary annoyance and nothing to worry about.

Troubleshooting

♦ If you feel worse in the 24 hours after your vibration session, try less time and/or frequency the next time. You can even rest a day, and then only vibrate two to three times per week. Another good way to slow down is to just sit next to the machine and put only your feet on the vibrating plate.

♦ It is highly recommended to incorporate a healthy diet and natural supplements to help lower inflammation and support healing in your body. See the detoxification section in Chapter 8 and my other books for other natural methods to add to your natural health program. The best results are achieved with a complete natural health program.

Advanced Program

Whole body vibration exercise is much more effective than conventional exercise. Workout times can be drastically shortened; you can accomplish the same results in 10–15 minutes that would take you 60 minutes with conventional exercise. (Note: This ratio applies only to the more powerful vibration machines I recommend such as the Power 1000. With gentler vibration, you're not getting the same type of intense exercise.)

This is true because WBV requires your body to constantly respond to the rapidly moving platform beneath you.

Four factors determine how effective and challenging your training sessions will be:

1. Frequency (rate of vibration)

2. Position or posture you assume

3. Amount of time you spend holding a given position

4. Amount of weight you are supporting on the plate (if you want a more challenging workout, hold additional exercise weights)

Static vs. Dynamic Exercises

It is important to note that exercises can be done statically or dynamically. Static exercises are more appropriate for beginners or when starting to rehabilitate from an injury. Dynamic exercises are great if you are looking to make an exercise more challenging.

♦ *Static exercise:* Holding a pose in a position without moving while the WBV machine is on

♦ *Dynamic exercise:* Moving while the WBV machine is on (doing push-ups, squats, etc.)

Progressive Training Plan

I recommend progressively phasing in the following elements to increase the difficulty of your workout. As your body adapts and grows stronger, you can continue to challenge yourself with these methods.

1. Extend the time of each exercise.

2. Reduce the rest period between exercises.

3. Increase the number of sets per exercise.

4. Perform exercises statically (standing still) and then dynamically (moving).

5. Add more challenging exercises.

6. Increase the frequency (Hz).

7. Incorporate unilateral exercises (perform exercises on one leg).

8. Incorporate holding increasing amounts of additional weight.

Thirty-Two Sample Exercise Positions, Massages, and Stretches

There are as many positions possible on the vibration plate as you can think of. Anything is fine. Experiment and see what feels good.

The following exercise positions are arranged by the areas of the body that they target, although some exercises target several areas of the body at the same time. First there are leg, hip, and buttock exercises; then arm, chest, and shoulder exercises; then abdominal and core exercises; and finally, balance poses, massages, and stretches. Within each body area grouping, the exercises are arranged from easier to harder.

The muscle-strengthening effect is greatest when holding the exercise positions, but even if you just stand on the vibrating plate, you will still be getting many benefits. Even though the exercises are grouped by the areas of your body you might wish to target, many of these exercises will also be using muscles all over your body. Some positions work on one side of the body at a time. When you do these, to keep things even, you should switch sides and do the position on the other side too. For pictures of many more suggested exercise positions, check out my poster available on Amazon and my website: www.BCVibrantHealth.com.

For static exercises, get into a position and hold it. For more intensive, dynamic exercises, you can move slowly in and out of the position.

Leg, Hip, and Buttock Exercises

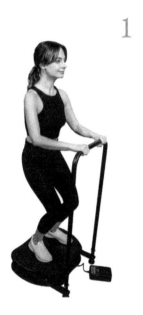

1

Beginner's position: Stand in a comfortable, balanced position with knees slightly flexed. If you enjoy the sensation of the vibration, you can straighten your legs, and more vibration will travel up through your bones to your entire body. If you don't like the vibration in your head, keep your knees bent. Hold onto a balance aid as needed. (Vibrant Health Ultimate Vibe machine with optional handle)

Deep squat: Position your feet slightly apart in the middle of the plate. Bend your knees about 80 degrees. Don't let your knees extend beyond your toes. Arch your back, keep your head up, and maintain balance. This position feels sort of like beginning to sit in a chair and then holding that position. (Vibrant Health Power 1000 machine)

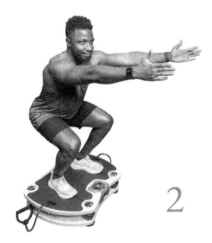

2

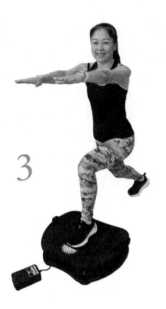

Lunge: Place one foot in the center of the plate, and bend your knee 60–90 degrees. Don't let your knee extend beyond your toes. Extend the opposite foot backward to the floor. Bending this back knee will make the exercise harder. You can hold a handlebar or other balance aid. For a more advanced and difficult position, put your arms straight out in front of you, and balance without holding on to anything. (Vibrant Health Ultimate Vibe machine)

One-legged squat: Stand in the middle of the plate. Lift and hold one leg behind you. Bend your other knee so you are in a squat position. Hold on to a balance aid as necessary. (Vibrant Health Power 1000 machine)

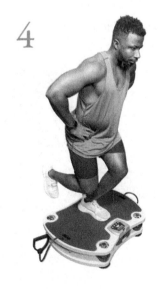

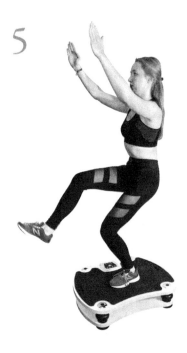

One-legged squat (advanced): Stand in the middle of the plate. Lift and hold one leg up in front of you with your foot stretched out. Bend your other knee so you are in a squat position. Hold your arms up high in front of you, and maintain balance. (Vibrant Health Power 1000 machine)

Pelvic bridge: Place feet on plate, slightly apart. Rest shoulders and head on the floor, and extend your arms along your sides. Lift your hips and hold in your stomach. (Vibrant Health Power 1000 machine)

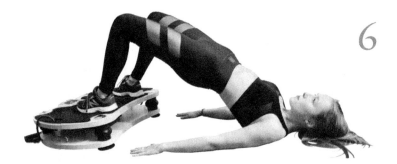

One-legged pelvic bridge: Place one foot at the center of the plate. Rest shoulders and head on the floor, and extend your arms along your sides. Extend your other leg up in line with your body or straight up into the air. Lift your hips, and hold in your stomach. (Vibrant Health Power 1000 machine)

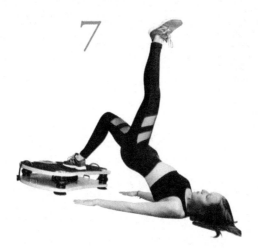

One-legged balance: Stand with one foot in the center of the plate. Bend that knee slightly. Stretch your other leg straight out behind you and your arms straight out in front of you. Maintain balance. (Vibrant Health Ultimate Vibe)

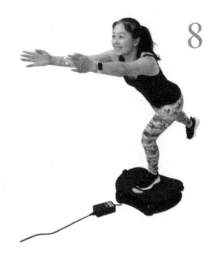

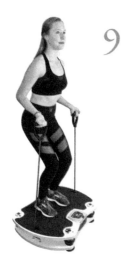

Slight squat arm exercise with straps: Stand on the plate with knees bent. Holding the stretchy straps, extend your arms in front of you with palms up and elbows bent. Pull up on the straps. (Vibrant Health Power 1000 machine)

Arm, Chest, and Shoulder Exercises

Lateral side raise: Stand upright on the plate, and with arms stretched out to the sides, pull up on the adjustable length cloth straps. (Vibrant Health Power 1000 machine)

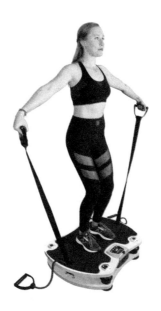

Back cross-strap pull: Stand on the plate in a slight squat. Hold each stretchy strap—palms down—in the hand opposite to the side the strap is on. Crossing the straps behind you, pull out to the side. (Vibrant Health Power 1000 machine)

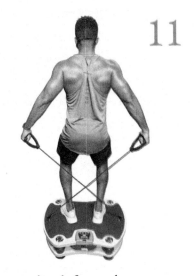

Beginner's push-up: Facing the plate, put your hands flat on the outer part of the plate. Rest your knees on the ground with your body straight from shoulders to knees. Tighten and hold your stomach in. With your shoulders over your hands, bend and straighten your elbows, moving your body up and down doing push-ups; or just bend your elbows and hold that position. (Vibrant Health Power 1000 machine)

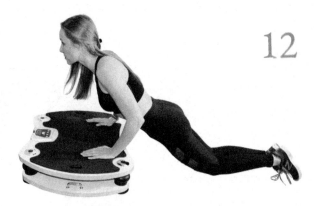

Advanced push-up: Facing the plate, put your hands flat on the outer edges, and keep your feet on the ground behind the plate. Keep your body straight from shoulders to feet, holding your stomach in. With your shoulders over your hands, bend and straighten your elbows, moving your body up and down doing push-ups; or just bend your elbows and hold that position. (Vibrant Health Ultimate Vibe)

13

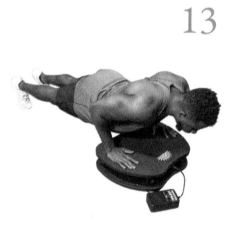

Shoulder press: Place your hands on the plate, fingers pointing forward. Align your shoulders above your hands. With your feet separated but close to the plate, stand on your toes if you can. To make this exercise more difficult, bend your elbows. This will increase the weight your arms and shoulders are supporting. (Vibrant Health Power 1000 machine)

14

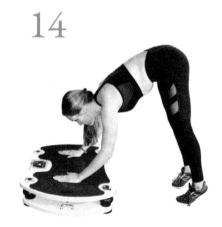

Triceps dip: With your back to the plate, place your hands at the front of the plate, shoulder width apart, pointing forward. Keeping your heels on the ground, bend your knees 90 degrees. Hold your waist in, and keep your back straight and your head up. Lower your buttocks by bending your elbows. Either hold that position or move up and down.

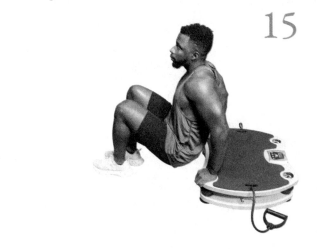

15

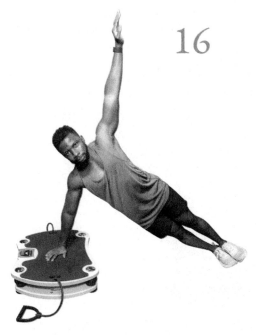

16

Side cross: Place one hand in the center of the plate with arm extended. Extend the other arm and hand straight upward. Extend legs in front of the plate, and keep hips in line with the legs and body, making a cross shape with your body. Alternate sides. (Vibrant Health Power 1000 machine)

Abdominal and Core Exercises

Easy abdominal: Lie with your back on the plate. Lift your head and touch the sides of your head with your hands. Lift your legs up, and bend your knees. Hold this position. The position will give you a back massage at the same time. (Vibrant Health Power 1000 machine)

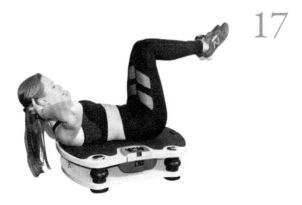

Easy sit-up: Sit sideways on the plate with your feet on the ground. With your arms outstretched or crossed, lean back, and then sit up straight again. Repeat this leaning back and sitting up straight again motion for 30 seconds. This exercise is an easy way to strengthen your abdominal muscles, which are essential for good posture and helping to prevent lower back pain. (Vibrant Health Ultimate Vibe)

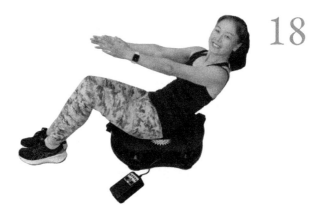

Sit-up: Sit sideways on the plate in a V-shaped position, leaning back and lifting your legs. The straighter the legs in this position, the harder it will be. Try it with bent knees at first. (Vibrant Health Power 1000 machine)

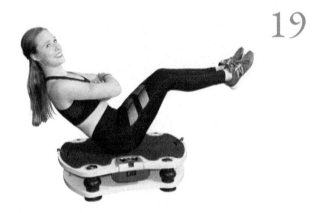

19

Diagonal crunch: Sit lengthwise on the plate. Bend one knee while straightening the other leg. Bring your hands to your ears, and bend your elbows. Touch your opposite elbow to the bent knee, and hold while tensing your abdominal muscles. (Vibrant Health Power 1000 machine)

20

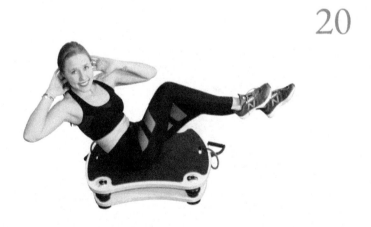

Pelvic stabilization: Place your hands on the center of the plate, slightly apart. Extend your arms with elbows slightly bent. Tense your abdominal muscles, and flatten and straighten your back. Rise up on your toes, and hold. (Vibrant Health Power 1000 machine)

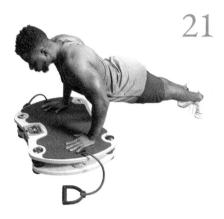

21

Pelvic stabilization 2: With your body facing up, place your hands on the front edge of the plate, shoulder width apart. Hold your body in a straight line from shoulders to heels. Tense your abdominal muscles, and flatten and straighten your back. (Vibrant Health Power 1000 machine)

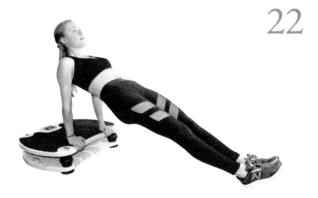

22

Plank: Position yourself face down with your toes on the floor and your forearms on the plate. Your elbows should be directly under your shoulders, and your hands should face forward. Tighten your abdominal muscles. Keep your back straight and your body in a straight line from head to toes—no sagging or bending. (Vibrant Health Ultimate Vibe)

23

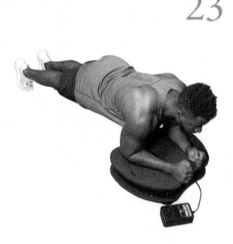

Reverse plank: Position yourself face down with your toes on the plate and your forearms on the floor. Your elbows should be directly under your shoulders, and your hands should face forward. Tighten your abdominal muscles. Keep your back straight and your body in a straight line from head to toes—no sagging or bending. (Vibrant Health Power 1000 machine)

24

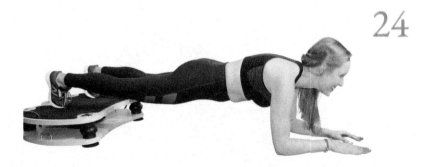

Balance, Stretching, and Massage Positions

Hamstring stretch: Stand on the center of the plate with your feet together, knees slightly bent. Bend at the waist, and grasp your ankles. This position stretches the hamstring muscles in the back of your upper legs. (Vibrant Health Power 1000 machine)

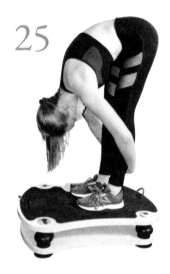

Adductor stretch: Stand in front of the plate, facing sideways. Place one foot on the plate toward the back so your leg is stretched. With your weight on the leg on the floor, bend that knee, and place your hands on your hips (or rest both hands on the bent knee). Slowly tense the inner thigh of the leg on the plate. This position stretches the muscles of your inner thigh. (Vibrant Health Power 1000 machine)

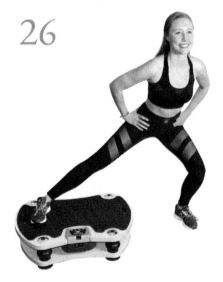

Back massage: Lie down with your back on the plate. Be sure to put a pillow under your head. DO NOT PUT YOUR HEAD DIRECTLY ON THE VIBRATING PLATE. Either lift your legs straight up above you, curl them in toward your stomach, or leave your feet on the floor—all these positions will give you different effects. (Vibrant Health Power 1000 machine)

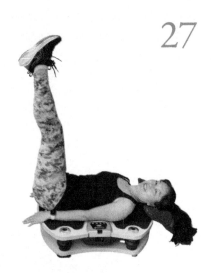

27

Glute massage: Sit on the plate with your hands on the plate and your back straight. Stretch your legs in front of you, and relax. (Vibrant Health Power 1000 machine)

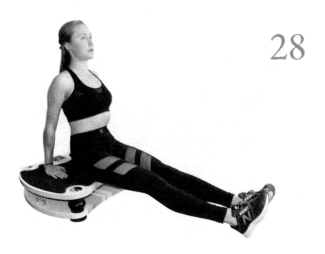

28

Hamstrings massage: Rest the backs of your thighs on the plate. Support your body weight on your hands. Hold your stomach in, and keep your back straight. (Vibrant Health Power 1000 machine)

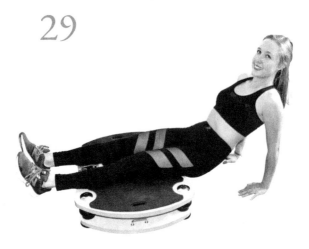

Quadriceps massage: Lie face down with your knees bent and your thighs on the plate. Support your body weight with your forearms, flatten your back, and relax. (Vibrant Health Power 1000 machine)

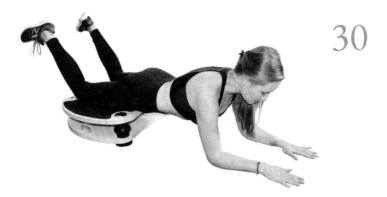

Tree pose (balance): Stand on one foot on the platform. Raise the other foot, and with bent knee, place that foot against the leg you are standing on. Raise your arms above your head with your fingertips touching, and balance. (Vibrant Health Ultimate Vibe with handle)

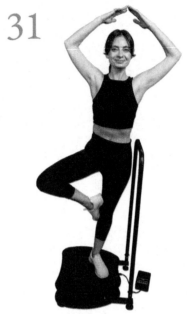

Calf massage: Place your calves on the plate, lie back on floor behind you, hands behind your head, and relax. This is super relaxing and a favorite position for many people. (Vibrant Health Power 1000 machine)

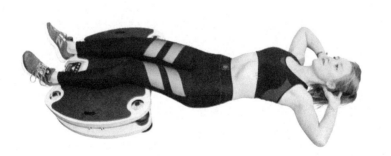

Vibrant Health Research Survey Summary

Effects of Whole Body Vibration Using the Vibrant Health Power 1000 in Retrospective Observational Survey[vii]

—Becky Chambers, BS, MEd.
and Jaswant Chaddha, MD, FACOG
(unpublished data, 2019)

Survey of People Who Use the Vibrant Health Power 1000 Machine

Specifications of the VH Power 1000 and Method of Use

♦ Type of vibration machine: Relatively gentle, single motor, vertical vibration (entire plate moves in the same direction, up and down, at the same time)

---

vii Becky Chambers and Jaswant Chaddha, "Effects of Whole Body Vibration Using the Vibrant Health Power 1000 in Retrospective Observational Survey," 2019, https://bcvibranthealth.com/wp-content/uploads/2019/06/Vibrant-Health-WBV-Survey2019.pdf.

- Frequency = 26–45 Hz (increasing in 1 Hz increments)
- Becky Chambers' "Slow & Gentle" method

Metrics of Study Respondents

- 53 respondents out of 187 surveys were sent out using HIPPA-protected online Survey Monkey website (28% response rate) in two weeks; no compensation was offered.

- 26% were 50–59 years of age, 62% were ages 60–80, 2% were over 90 years of age. A total of 90% of respondents were over age 50.

- 58% female, 42% male

- 80% in average, good, or excellent health (self-rating)

- Most reported eating a healthy diet and taking few to no drugs.

- 55% had their machine one to two years, 43% for one to twelve months.

- Most had never used a vibration machine before.

- 64% reported following Becky's "Slow & Gentle" plan for starting WBV; 54% said this approach was important to them.

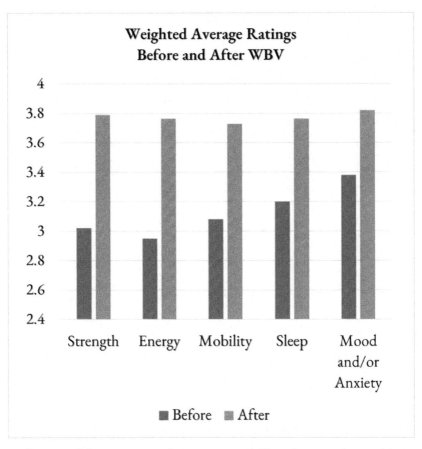

Five modalities—strength, energy, mobility, sleep, and mood/anxiety—were self-rated on a scale of 1 to 5, with "1" being weak/low/poor and "5" being very strong/high or excellent.

Improvements with WBV

Significant improvements were seen in:

Strength	25%
Energy	28%
Mobility	20%
Sleep	17%
Mood	14%

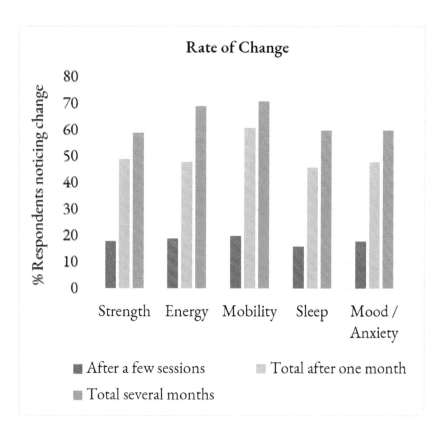

All modalities improved rapidly: strength, energy, mobility, sleep, and mood/anxiety.

♦ 15–20% improved after a few WBV sessions
♦ 45–60% total within a month
♦ 60–70% total within several months

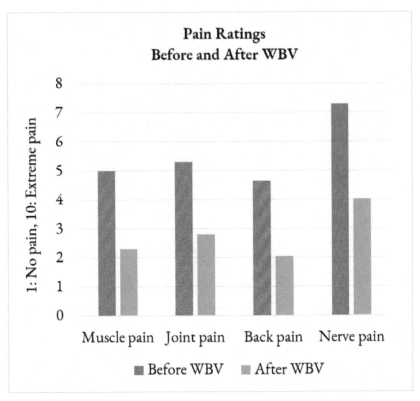

Thirty-nine respondents reported having muscle, joint, back, or nerve pain when they started vibrating. For all those reporting pain at the beginning of their WBV program, the average reported pain reduction was 31%. Of those who reported an improvement in pain (74% of the 39 people who reported pain), their average reported drop in pain levels was 52%. Twenty percent of the thirty-nine respondents also reduced their pain medications after beginning WBV or switched to less powerful meds while reporting less pain. Most respondents took no pain medications.

Joints all over the body improved, especially knee joints.

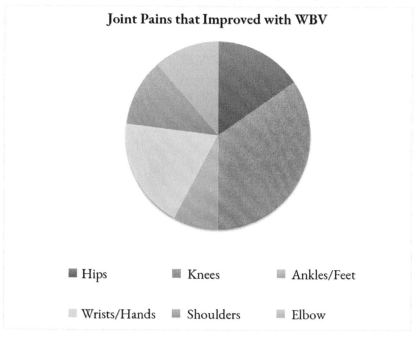

Pain relief was rapid for muscle, joint, back, and nerve pain. Most people whose pain improved noticed this improvement within weeks of beginning their WBV program.

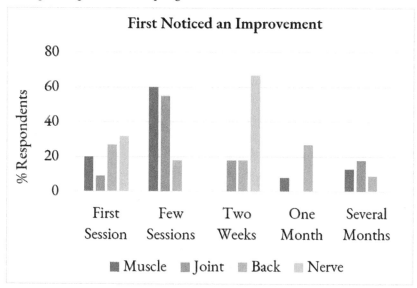

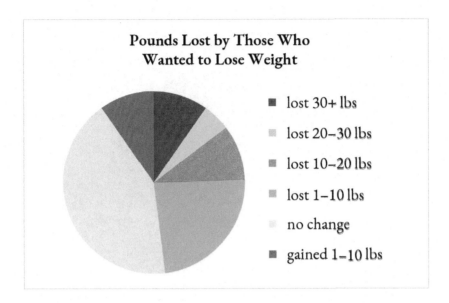

Pounds Lost by Those Who Wanted to Lose Weight

- lost 30+ lbs
- lost 20–30 lbs
- lost 10–20 lbs
- lost 1–10 lbs
- no change
- gained 1–10 lbs

Almost half of those who wanted to lose weight did lose weight, ranging from a few pounds to over thirty pounds. Virtually all of the respondents (98%) were not taking weight-loss supplements or medications. Most followed healthy, low carb diet regimens, and 86% did not change their diets. There was very little change in the amount of type of other exercise for most respondents.

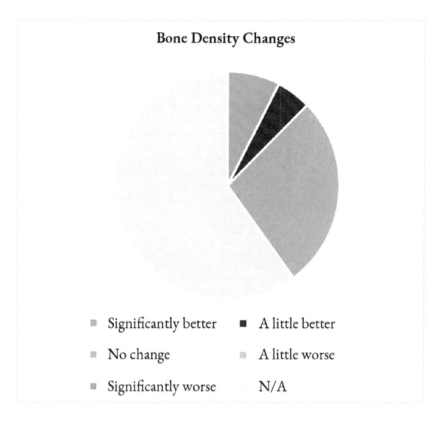

Bone density:

♦ 40% of respondents increased their bone density or did not lose bone density.

♦ 0% of respondents lost bone density.

♦ Considering that a large percentage of the respondents in this survey either already had osteopenia or osteoporosis, or were at high risk of developing low bone density, these results are excellent, indicating a reversal or interruption of the normal progression of this disease for 40% or more of the survey respondents.

♦ 60% answered Not Applicable (N/A). Most likely, many respondents had not used their machines long enough to have had a recent bone-density test and therefore were not able to answer this question.

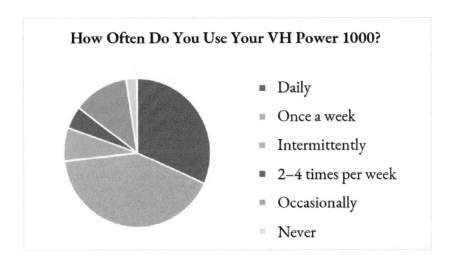

How Often Do You Use Your VH Power 1000?

- Daily
- Once a week
- Intermittently
- 2–4 times per week
- Occasionally
- Never

Seventy-three percent of respondents use their vibration machine at least two to four times per week. Only 8% use their machine occasionally or never.

WBV Contraindications

It is always advisable to consult with your physician before starting any exercise program. Ongoing research in the field of whole body vibration (WBV) indicates that it can lower inflammation and that many people can benefit from this form of exercise. However, if you suffer from any of the following contraindications, it is imperative that you discuss WBV therapy with your physician before beginning any training program with WBV equipment.

NOTE REGARDING LOW INTENSITY VIBRATION (LIV)

According to the FDA, there are no contraindication for the extremely gentle form of vibration called low intensity vibration (LIV). However, I would still recommend caution with LIV with certain very sensitive conditions such as epilepsy controlled with medications, severe acute migraines, vertigo, retinal detachment issues, recently broken bones, joint replacements, and other conditions listed in the Absolute Contraindications category.

Relative Contraindications: These conditions, with special care and treatment, can sometimes not be a hindrance to and may even benefit from WBV.

Please do not use a WBV device without first getting approval from your doctor if you have any of the following relative contraindications:

- Pregnancy
- Epilepsy (very mild and not needing to be controlled with medications)
- Minor migraines (mild, infrequent, and not needing to be controlled by medication)
- Gallstones, kidney stones, bladder stones (WBV can help small stones move out of the body, but large ones may get stuck, potentially leading to severe problems.)
- Articular rheumatism, arthrosis
- Acute rheumatoid arthritis
- Heart failure
- Cardiac dysrhythmia
- Cardiac disorders (post-myocardial infarction [heart attack])
- Metal or synthetic implants (e.g., pacemaker, artificial cardiac valves, recent stents, or brain implants)
- Chronic back pain after fracture, disc disorders, or spondylosis.
- Severe diabetes mellitus with peripheral vascular disease or neuropathy
- Tumors (excluding metastases in the musculoskeletal system)
- Spondylolisthesis (a misalignment front to back of the vertebrae) without gliding
- Movement disorders: Parkinson's disease, MS, cerebral palsy, and others
- Chondromalacia of the joints of the lower extremities, osteonecrosis
- Arterial circulation disorders

- Venous insufficiency with *ulcus cruris*

- Morbus Sudeck Stadium II (or complex regional pain syndrome [CRPS])

- Lymphatic edema

- Postoperative wounds

Absolute Contraindications—meaning do not use a WBV device at all (with the possible exception of LIV*) if you have any of the following or if you have any concerns about your physical health!

> *NOTE: For conditions in which absolutely no vibration can be tolerated—broken bones, recent joint replacements and implants, and others—be aware that vibration will travel through wooden floors. In these cases, do not sit or stand next to a powerful vibrating plate. A cement floor should be safe since very little vibration will transmit through cement.*

It is likely that LIV can be safely used with (and may even benefit) many of these conditions, but please talk to your doctor before using any vibration with these conditions.

- Acute inflammations, infections, and/or fever

- Large gallstones, kidney stones, bladder stones (large enough to potentially get stuck in narrow tubes on the way out of your body)

- Acute arthropathy or arthrosis (such as an acute arthritis attack from an infectious or autoimmune disease)

- Joint replacements: you must wait six months after a joint replacement before using WBV. After that time, WBV is okay; the vibration will then improve the bond of bone to metal or other synthetic material.

- Bone fractures: for simple bone fractures, after six weeks it is okay to use WBV. For complex fractures or those involving implanted metal plates or screws, you must wait eight to twelve weeks before using WBV. Please consult with your doctor regarding your particular situation.

- Acute migraine

- Acute or severe epilepsy (needs to be controlled with medication)

- Retinal detachment (or a high risk of retinal detachment)

- Fresh (surgical) wounds

- Implants of the spine (spinal fusions are not a contraindication as long as they are healed)

- Acute or chronic deep vein thrombosis or other thrombotic afflictions

- Acute disc-related problems, spondylolysis (stress fracture of the vertebrae), gliding spondylolisthesis, or fractures

- Severe osteoporosis with bmd less than 70 mg/ml (T-scores less than −3.9)

- Spasticity (after stroke, spinal cord lesion, etc.)

- Morbus Sudeck Stadium I (CRPS I)

- Tumors with metastases in the musculoskeletal system

- Vertigo or positional dizziness

- Acute myocardial infarction

Additional Research Studies

For more information, go to http://www.ncbi.nlm.nih.gov/ pubmed or scholar.google.com and use the search string "whole body vibration" to find hundreds of other research studies.

Brain Synchronization

Abraha, Iosief., Fabiana Trotta, Joseph M. Rimland, Alfonso Cruz-Jentoft, Isabel Lozano-Montoya, Roy L. Soiza, Valentina Pierini, Paolo Dessi Fulgheri, Fabrizia Lattanzio, Denis O'Mahony, and Antonio Cherubini. "Efficacy of Non-Pharmacological Interventions to Prevent and Treat Delirium in Older Patients: A Systematic Overview. The SENATOR Project ONTOP Series." *PLoS One* 10, no. 6 (2015): e1023090. https://doi.org/10.1371/journal.pone.0123090.

Danilenko, K. V., and I. A. Ivanova. "Dawn Simulation vs. Bright Light in Seasonal Affective Disorder: Treatment Effects and Subjective Preference." *Journal of Affective Disorders* 180 (July 15, 2015): 87–9. https://doi.org/10.1016/j.jad.2015.03.055.

da Silva, Vernon Furtado, Alair Pedro Ribeiro, Veruska Andrea dos Santos, Antonio Egidio Nardi, Anna Lucia Spear King, and Mauricio Rocha Calomeni. "Stimulation by Light and Sound: Therapeutics Effects in Humans: Systematic Review." *Clinical Practice & Epidemiology in Mental Health* 11 (June 26, 2015): 150–4. https://doi.org/10.2174/1745017901511010150.

Petrovsky, Darina, Pamela Z. Cacchione, and Maureen George. "Review of the Effect of Music Interventions on Symptoms of Anxiety and Depression in Older Adults with Mild Dementia." *International Psychogeriatrics* 27, no. 10 (October 2015): 1–10. https://doi.org/10.1017/S1041610215000393.

Raglio, Alfred, Caterina Galandra, Luisella Sibilla, Fabrizio Esposito, Francesca Gaeta, Francesco Di Salle, Luca Moro, Irene Carne, Stefano Bastianello, Maurizia Baldi, and Marcello Imbriani. "Effects of Active Music Therapy on the Normal Brain: fMRI Based Evidence." *Brain Imaging and Behavior* 10, no. 1

(March 2016): 182–6. https://doi.org/10.1007/s11682-015-9380-x.

Schwartz, Richard S., and Jacqueline Olds. "The Psychiatry of Light." *Harvard Review of Psychiatry* 23, no. 3 (May/June 2015): 188–94. https://doi.org/10.1097/HRP.0000000000000078.

Shealy, C. N. "The Reality of EEG and Neurochemical Responses to Photostimulation: Part I." In *Light Years Ahead: The Illustrated Guide to Full Spectrum and Colored Light in Mindbody Healing,* edited by Brian Breiling et al. Berkeley: Celestial Arts Press, 1996.

————. "The Reality of EEG and Neurochemical Responses to Photostimulation: Part II." In *Light Years Ahead: The Illustrated Guide to Full Spectrum and Colored Light in Mindbody Healing,* edited by Brian Breiling et al. Berkeley: Celestial Arts Press, 1996.

————, R. K. Cady, D. C. Veehoff, M. Burnetti-Atwell, R. Houston, and R. H. Cox. "Effects of Color Photostimulation upon Neurochemicals and Neurohormones." *Journal of Neurological and Orthopaedic Medicine and Surgery* 17, no. 1 (1996): 95–6.

————, Timothy L. Smith, P. Thomlinson, and W. Tiller. "A Double-Blind EEG Response Test for a Supposed Electromagnetic Field-Neutralizing Device. Part I: Via the Clinician Expertise Procedure." *Subtle Energies & Energy Medicine Journal Archives* 9, no. 3, 231–45.

Sun J., and W. Chen. "Music Therapy for Coma Patients: Preliminary Results." *European Review for Medical and Pharmacological Sciences* 19, no. 7 (April 2015): 1209–18.

Harmful Consequences

Diemen, A. "Vibration Training: Mechanisms and Possible Mechanisms Relating to Structural Adaptations and Acute Effects." *Sweelinkplein Nederland* 1 (2002): 21–34.

Kelderman, Janneke. "The Power Plate: A New Application in Physical Therapy?" Groningen, 2001.

Kleinöder, H., J. Ziegler, C. Bosse, and J. Mester. "Safety Considerations in Vibration Training." Institute of Training and Movement Science, German Sport University Cologne.

Stoppani, Jim. "Shake, Rattle, and Grow: The Science and Application of Vibration Training."

Meditation

Tlalka, Stephany. "Meditation Is the Fastest Growing Health Trend in America." *Health* (December 11, 2018).

Zeidan, Fadel, and David R. Vago. "Mindfulness Meditation-Based Pain Relief: A Mechanistic Account." *Annals of the New York Academy of Sciences* 1373, no. 1 (June 2016): 114–27. https://doi.org/10.1111/nyas.13153.

Mind-Body Immune

System Connection

Al-Ayadhi, Laila Y. "Neurohormonal Changes in Medical Students during Academic Stress." *Annals of Saudi Medicine* 25, no. 1 (January–February 2005): 36–40. https://doi.org/10.5144/0256-4947.2005.36.

D'Acquisto, Fulvio. "Affective Immunology: Where Emotions and the Immune Response Converge." *Dialogues in Clinical Neuroscience* 19, no. 1 (March 2017): 9–19.

MacDonald, Catherine M. "A Chuckle a Day Keeps the Doctor Away: Therapeutic Humor and Laughter." *Journal of Psychosocial Nursing and Mental Health Services* 42, no. 3 (March 2004): 18–25.

Vedhara, K., N. K. Cox, G. K. Wilcock, P. Perks, M. Hunt, S. Anderson, S. L. Lightman, and N. M. Shanks. "Chronic Stress in Elderly Carers of Dementia Patients and Antibody Response to Influenza Vaccination." *The Lancet* 353, no. 9153 (February 1999): 627–31. https://doi.org/10.1016/S0140-6736(98)06098-X.

Performance

Bosco, Carmelo, M. Cardinale, Roberto Colli, József Tihanyi, Priya S. von Duvillard, and Atko Viru. "The Influence of Whole Body Vibration on the Mechanical Behaviour of Skeletal Muscle." *Clinical Physiology* 19 (1999): 183–7.

———, Marco Cardinale., and Olga Tsarpela. "Influence of Vibration on Mechanical Power and Electromyogram Activity in Human Arm Flexor Muscles." *European Journal of Applied Physiology* 79, no. 4 (1999): 306–11.

———, Marco Cardinale, Olga Tsarpela, and Elio Locatelli. "New Trends in Training Science: The Use of Vibrations for Enhancing Performance." *New Studies in Athletics* 4, no. 14 (1999): 55–62.

————, Carmelo, Roberto Colli, E. Introini, Marco Cardinale, Olga Tsarpela, A. Madella, József Tihanyi, and Atko Viru. "Adaptive Responses of Human Skeletal Muscle to Vibration Exposure." *Clinical Physiology* 19, no. 2 (1999): 183–7.

de Ruiter, C. J., R. M. van der Linden, M. J. A. van der Zijden, A. P. Hollander, and A. de Haan. "Short-Term Effects of Whole-Body Vibration on Maximal Voluntary Isometric Knee Extensor Force and Rate of Force Rise." *European Journal of Applied Physiology* 88, no. 4–5 (2003): 472–5.

Hinman, Martha R. "Whole Body Vibration: A New Exercise Approach." Department of Physical Therapy, The University of Texas Medical Branch.

Humphries, B., and G. Warman. "The Assessment of Vibromyographical Signals in the Time and Frequency Domains during a Fatigue Protocol." The School of Health and Human Performance, Central Queensland University.

Issurin, V. B., and G. Tenenbaum. "Acute and Residual Effects of Vibratory Stimulation on Explosive Strength in Elite and Amateur Athletes." *Journal of Sports Sciences* 17, no. 3 (March 1999): 177–82.

Nishihihira, Y., T. Iwasaki, A. Hatta, T. Wasaka, T. Kaneda, K. Kuroiwa, S. Akiyama, T. Kida, and K. S. Ryol. "Effect of Whole Body Vibration Stimulus and Voluntary Contraction on Motoneuron Pool." Japan Society of Exercise and Sports Physiology, Tsukuba (2002): 83–86.

Rittweger, J., G. Beller, and D. Felsenberg. "Acute Physiological Effects of Exhaustive Whole-Body Vibration Exercise in Man." *Clinical Physiology* 20, no. 2 (March 2000): 134–42.

————, J. Ehrig, K. Just, M. Mutschelknauss, K. A. Kirsch, and D. Felsenberg. "Oxygen Uptake in Whole-Body Vibration Exercise: Influence of Vibration Frequency, Amplitude, and External Load." *International Journal of Sports Medicine* 23, no. 6 (August 2002): 428–32.

————, Marcus Mutschelknauss, and Dieter Felsenberg. "Acute Changes in Neuromuscular Excitability after Exhaustive Whole Body Vibration Exercise as Compared to Exhaustion by Squatting Exercise." *Clinical Physiology and Functional Imaging* 23, no. 2 (March 2003): 81–6.

————, H. Schiessl, and D. Felsenberg. "Oxygen Uptake during Whole-Body Vibration Exercise: Comparison with Squatting as a Slow Voluntary Movement." *European Journal of Applied Physiology* 86, no. 2 (December 2001): 169–73.

Torvinen, Saila, Pekka Kannus, Harri Sievänen, Tero A. H. Järvinen, Matti Pasanen, Saija Kontulainen, Teppo L. N. Järvinen, Markku Järvinen, Pekka Oja, and Ilkka Vuori. "Effect of Four-Month Vertical Whole Body Vibration on Performance and Balance." *Medicine and Science in Sports and Exercise* 34, no. 9 (2002): 1523–8.

————. "Effect of Vibration Exposure on Muscular Performance and Body Balance: Randomized Cross-Over Study." *Clinical Physiology and Functional Imaging* 22, no. 2 (March 2002): 145–52.

Quality of Life

Hormonal Response

Cardinale, Marcos. "The Effects of Vibration on Human Performance and Hormonal Profile." PhD Thesis, The Semmelweis University Doctoral School, Faculty of Physical Education and Sport Sciences, Budapest 2002.

————, and Jon Lim. "Electromyography Activity of Vastus Lateralis Muscle during Whole-Body Vibrations of Different Frequencies." *Journal of Strength and Conditioning Research* 17, no. 3 (August 2003): 621–4.

Carroll, Timothy J., Stephan Riek, and Richard G. Carson. "The Sites of Neural Adaptation Induced by Resistance Training in Humans." *Journal of Physiology* 544, no.2 (October 2002): 641–52.

Delecluse, Christophe, Machteld Roelants, and Sabine Verschueren. "Strength Increase after Whole Body Vibration Compared with Resistance Training." *Medicine and Science in Sports and Exercise* 35, no. 6 (June 2003): 1033–41.

Blood Circulation

Kerschan-Schindl, K., S. Grampp, C. Henk, H. Resch, E. Preisinger, V. Fialka-Moser, and H. Imhof. "Whole-Body Vibration Exercise Leads to Alterations in Muscle Blood Volume." *Clinical Physiology* 21, no. 3 (May 2001): 377–82.

Pain Management

Brumagne, S., P. Cordo, R. Lysens, S. Verschueren, and S. Swinnen. "The Role of Paraspinal Muscle Spindles in Lumbosacral Position Sense in Individuals with and without Low Back Pain." *Spine* 25, no. 8 (2000): 989–94.

Gianutsos, J. G., J. H. Ahn, E. F. Richter, B. B. Grynbaum, and H. G. Thistle. "The Effects of Whole Body Vibration on Reflex-Induced Standing in Persons with Chronic and Acute Spinal Cord Injury." *5th International Congress of Physical Medicine and Rehabilitation*, Athens, 2000.

Bone Density

Bruyere, Olivier, Marc=Antoine Wuidart, Elio Di Plama, and Jean-Yves Reginster. "Controlled Whole Body Vibrations Improve Health Related Quality of Life in Elderly Patients." American College of Rheumatology. (October 23–28, 2003): Abstract 1271.

Falempin, M., and S. F. In-Albon. "Influence of Brief Daily Tendon Vibration on Rat Soleus Muscle in a Non-Weight-Bearing Situation." *Journal of Applied Physiology* 87, no. 1 (July 1999): 3–9.

Flieger, J., T. Karachalios, L. Khaldi, P. Raptou, and G. Lyritis. "Mechanical Stimulation in the Form of Vibration Prevents Postmenopausal Bone Loss in Ovariectomized Rats." *Calcified Tissue International* 63, no. 6 (December 1998): 510–4.

Rubin, Clinton, Malcolm Pope, J. Chris Fritton, Marianne Magnusson, Tommy Hansson, and Kenneth McLeod. "Transmissibility of 15-Hertz to 35-Hertz Vibrations to the Human Hip and Lumbar Spine: Determining the Physiologic Feasibility of Delivering Low-Level Anabolic Mechanical Stimuli to Skeletal Regions at Greatest Risk of Fracture because of Osteoporosis." *Spine* 28, no. 23 (December 2003): 2621–7.

———, Robert Recker, Diane Cullen, John Ryaby, Joan McCabe, and Kenneth McLeod. "Prevention of Postmenopausal Bone Loss by a Low-Magnitude, High-Frequency Mechanical Stimuli: A Clinical Trial Assessing Compliance, Efficacy, and Safety." *Journal of Bone and Mineral Research* 19, no. 3 (March 2004): 343–51.

———, S. A. Turner, S. Bain, C. Mallinckrodt, and K. McLeod. "Anabolism: Low Mechanical Signals Strengthen Long Bones." *Nature* 412 (2001): 603–604.

———, Gang Xu, and Stefan Judex. "The Anabolic Activity of Bone Tissue, Suppressed by Disuse, Is Normalized by Brief Exposure to Extremely Low Magnitude Mechanical Stimuli." *FASEB Journal* 15 (October 1, 2001): 2225–9.

Schiessel, H., H. M. Frost, and W. S. Jee. "Estrogen and Bone-Muscle Strength and Mass Relationships." *Bone* 22, no. 1 (January 1998): 1–6.

van Loon, Jack J. W. A., J. Paul Veldhuijzen, and Elizabeth H. Burger. "Bone and Space Flight: An Overview." In *Biological and Medical Research in Space,* edited by David Moore, Peter Bie, and Heinz Oser, 259–299. Berlin Heidelberg: Springer-Verlag, 1996.

Verschueren, Sabine M. P., Machteld Roelants, Christophe Delecluse, Stephan Swinnen, Dirk Vanderschueren, and Steven Boonen. "Effect of 6-Month

Whole Body Vibration Training on Hip Density, Muscle Strength, and Postural Control in Postmenopausal Women: A Randomized Controlled Pilot Study." *Journal of Bone and Mineral Research* 19, no. 3 (March 2004): 352–9.

Metabolism

Frank, H., B. Moos, A. Kaufmann, and H. A. Herber. "Anti-Cellulite Untersuchung. Sanaderm, Fach klinik fur Hautkrankheiten." *Allergologie* (2003): 1–35.

Flexibility/Mobility/Balance

Ishitake, T., Y. Miyazaki, H. Ando, and T. Mataka. *International Archives of Occupational and Environmental Health* 72, no. 7 (October 1999): 469–74.

Miyamoto, K., S. Mori, S. Tsuji, S. Tanaka, M. Kawamoto, T. Mashiba, S. Komatsubara, T. Akiyama, J. Kawanishi, and H. Norimatsu. "Whole-Body Vibration Exercise in the Elderly People." *IBMS-JSBMR* (2003): Abstract P506.

Rauch, F., and J. Rittweger. "What Is New in Neuro-Musculoskeletal Interactions?" *Journal of Musculoskeletal Neuron Interactions* 2, no. 5 (2002): 1–5.

Rogan, Slavko, Roger Hilfiker, Kaspar Herren, Lorenz Radlinger, and Eling D. de Bruin. "Effects of Whole-Body Vibration on Postural Control in Elderly: A Systematic Review and Meta-Analysis." *BMC Geriatrics* 11, no. 72 (2011).

Runge, M. "Therapiemöglichkeiten bei Harninkontinenz; überwinden des Tabu." *Der Hausarzt* 2 (2002): 56–61.

———, G. Rehfeld, and E. Reswick. "Balance Training and Exercise in Geriatric Patients." *Journal of Musculoskeletal Interactions* 1, no. 1 (2000): 61–5.

von der Heide, S., G. Emons, R. Hilgers, and V. Viereck. "Effect on Muscles of Mechanical Vibrations Produced by the Galileo 2000 in Combination with Physical Therapy in Treating Female Stress Urinary Incontinence." *International Continence Society 33rd Annual Meeting*, Florence, Italy, October 5–9, 2003.

Resources and Additional Reading

Resources

Becky Chambers, Naturopath, BS, MEd
Vibrant Health
www.bcvibranthealth.com

Candida Yeast

Boroch, Ann. *The Candida Cure: The 90-Day Program To Balance Your Gut, Beat Candida, and Restore Vibrant Health.* New York: HarperCollins, 2018.

Chaitow, Leon. *Candida Albicans: Could Yeast Be Your Problem?* Rochester, VT: Healing Arts Press, 1998.

Crook, William G. *The Yeast Connection: A Medical Breakthrough.* Berkeley, CA: Crown Publishing Group, 1994

Trowbridge, John Parks, and Morton Walker. *The Yeast Syndrome.* New York: Bantam Books, 1985.

Wunderlich, Ray Jr. *The Candida-Yeast Syndrome.* New York: McGraw-Hill, 1998.

Physical Therapy

Albasini, Alfio, Martin Krause, and Ingo Volker Rembitzki. *Using Whole Body Vibration in Physical Therapy and Sport: Clinical Practice and Treatment Exercises.* Edinburgh; New York: Churchill Livingstone/Elsevier, 2010.

Endnotes

Chapter 1

1. D. J. Cochrane, "Vibration Exercise: The Potential Benefits," *International Journal of Sports Medicine* 32, no. 2 (2011): 75–99, https://doi.org.10.1055/s-0030-1268010.

2. Shanawaz Anwer et al., "Effect of Whole Body Vibration Training on Quadriceps Muscle Strength in Individuals with Knee Osteoarthritis: A Systematic Review and Meta-Analysis," *Physiotherapy* 102, no. 2 (June 2016): 145–51, https://doi.org.10.1016/j.physio.2015.10.004.

3. Becky Chambers and Jaswant Chaddha, "Effects of Whole Body Vibration Using the Vibrant Health Power 1000 in Retrospective Observational Survey," unpublished data (2019), www.BCVibrantHealth.com.

Chapter 2

4. Jack C. Yu et al., "Whole Body Vibration-Induced Omental Macrophage Polarization and Fecal Microbiome Modification in a Murine Model," *International Journal of Molecular Science* 20, no. 13 (June 26, 2019): 3125, https://doi.org/10.3390/ijms20133125.

5. Ning Song et al., "Whole Body Vibration Triggers a Change in the Mutual Shaping State of Intestinal Microbiota and Body's Immunity," *Frontiers in Bioengineering and Biotechnology* (November 2019), https://doi.org/10.3389/fbioe.2019.00377.

6. Gabriel M. Pagnotti et al., "Combating Osteoporosis and Obesity with Exercise: Leveraging Cell Mechanosensitivity," *Nature Reviews Endocrinology* 15 (2019): 339–55, https://doi.org/10.1038/s41574-019-0170-1.

7. Carmelo Bosco et al., "Hormonal Responses to Whole-Body Vibration in Men," *European Journal of Applied Physiology* 81, no. 6 (2000): 449–54, https://doi.org/10.1007/s004210050067.

8. Matteo Zago et al., "Whole-Body Vibration Training in Obese Subjects: A Systematic Review," *PLoS One* 13, no. 9 (September 2018): e0202866, https://doi.org/10.1371/journal.pone.0202866.

9. Chiara Milanese et al., "Ten-Week Whole-Body Vibration Training Improves Body Composition and Muscle Strength in Obese Women," *International Journal of Medical Sciences* 10, no. 3 (2013): 307–311, https://doi.org/10.7150/ijms.5161.

10. Moushira Erfan Zaki, "Effects of Whole Body Vibration and Resistance

Training on Bone Mineral Density and Anthropometry in Obese Post-menopausal Women," *Journal of Osteoporosis* (2014): 702589, https://doi.org/10.1155/2014/702589.

11. Dirk Vissers et al., "Effect of Long-Term Whole Body Vibration Training on Visceral Adipose Tissue: A Preliminary Report," *Obesity Facts* 3, no. 2 (2010): 93–100, https://doi.org/10.1159/000301785.

12. Asako Miyaki et al., "The Addition of Whole-Body Vibration to a Life-style Modification on Arterial Stiffness in Overweight and Obese Women," *Artery Research* 6, no. 2 (June 2012): 85–91, https://doi.org/10.1016/j.artres.2012.01.006.

13. Jose Carmelo Adsuar et al., "Vibratory Exercise Training Effects on Weight in Sedentary Women with Fibromyalgia," *International Journal of Medicine and Science in Physical Education and Sport* 13, no. 60 (2013): 295–305, https://www.researchgate.net/publication/286411646_Vibratory_exercise_training_effects_on_weight_in_sedentary_women_with_fibromyalgia.

14. Borja Sañudo et al., "Whole Body Vibration Training Improves Leg Blood Flow and Adiposity in Patients with Type 2 Diabetes Mellitus," *European Journal of Applied Physiology* 113, no. 9 (2013): 2245–52, https://doi.org/10.1007/s00421-013-2654-3.

15. A. Bellia et al., "Effects of Whole Body Vibration Plus Diet on Insulin-Resistance in Middle-Aged Obese Subjects," *International Journal of Sports Medicine* 35, no. 6 (2014): 511–16, https://doi.org/10.1055/s-0033-1354358.

16. Dirk Vissers et al., "Effect of Long-Term Whole Body Vibration Training on Visceral Adipose Tissue: A Preliminary Report," *Obesity Facts* 3, no.2 (2010): 93–100, https://doi.org/10.1159/000301785.

17. S. Mohammad Alavinia, Maryam Omidvar, and B. Catharine Craven, "Does Whole Body Vibration Therapy Assist in Reducing Fat Mass or Treating Obesity in Healthy Overweight and Obese Adults? A Systematic Review and Meta-Analyses," *Disability and Rehabilitation* 43, no. 14 (2021): 1935–47, https://doi.org/10.1080/09638288.2019.1688871.

18. Alavinia, "Does Whole Body Vibration Therapy Assist in Reducing Fat Mass?"

19. Chambers and Chaddha, "Effects of Whole Body Vibration Using the Vibrant Health Power 1000."

20. Gina Kolata, "Low Buzz May Give Mice Better Bones and Less Fat," *The New York Times* (October 30, 2007), https://www.nytimes.com/2007/10/30/health/research/30bone.html?_r=1.

21. Gabriel M. Pagnotti et al., "Combating Osteoporosis and Obesity with Exercise: Leveraging Cell Mechanosensitivity," *Nature Reviews Endocrinology* 15 (2019): 339–55, https://doi.org/10.1038/s41574-019-0170-1.

22. Kris Gunnars, "Does All Disease Begin in Your Gut? The Surprising Truth," Healthline, February 27, 2019, https://www.healthline.com/nutrition/does-all-disease-begin-in-the-gut.

23. Meghan E. McGee-Lawrence et al., "Whole-Body Vibration Mimics the Metabolic Effects of Exercise in Male Leptin Receptor–Deficient Mice," *Endocrinology* 158, no. 5 (2017): 1160–71, https://doi.org/10.1210/en.2016-1250.

24. Hongyu Yin et al., "Whole Body Vibration Therapy: A Novel Potential Treatment for Type 2 Diabetes Mellitus," *SpringerPlus* 4 (2015): 578, https://doi.org/10.1186/s40064-015-1373-0.

25. Mitch Leslie, "Good Vibrations: A Bit of Shaking Can Burn Fat, Combat Diabetes," *Science* (March 15, 2017), https://doi.org/10.1126/science.aal0919.

26. Yu et al., "Whole Body Vibration-Induced Omental Macrophage Polarization."

27. Hongyu Yin et al., "Whole Body Vibration Therapy."

28. Yameena Jawed et al., "Whole-Body Vibration Training Increases Stem/Progenitor Cell Circulation Levels and May Attenuate Inflammation," *Military Medicine* 185, suppl. no. 1 (January–February 2020): 404–12, https://doi.org/10.1093/milmed/usz247.

29. Zago et al., "Whole-Body Vibration Training in Obese Subjects."

30. "Good Vibrations: A New Treatment under Study by NASA-Funded Doctors Could Reverse Bone Loss Experienced by Astronauts in Space," NASA, November 2, 2001, https://web.archive.org/web/20020209180125/http://science.nasa.gov/headlines/y2001/ast02nov_1.htm.

Chapter 3

31. "Good Vibrations: A New Treatment under Study by NASA-Funded Doctors."

32. Kolata, "Low Buzz May Give Mice Better Bones and Less Fat."

33. A. Prioreschi et al., "Whole Body Vibration Increases Hip Bone Mineral Density in Road Cyclists," *International Journal of Sports Medicine* 33, no. 8 (August 2012): 593–99, https://doi.org/10.1055/s-0032-1301886.

34. Prioreschi, "In Patients with Established RA, Positive Effects."

35. Kate Ward et al., "Low Magnitude Mechanical Loading Is Osteogenic in Children with Disabling Conditions," *Journal of Bone and Mineral Research* 19, no. 3 (2009): 360–69, https://doi.org/10.1359/JBMR.040129.

36. Elena Marín-Cascales et al., "Whole-Body Vibration Training and Bone Health in Postmenopausal Women: A Systematic Review and Meta-Analysis," *Medicine* 97, no. 34 (August 2018): e11918, https://doi.org/10.1097/MD.0000000000011918.

37. Marin-Cascales et al., "Whole-Body Vibration Training and Bone Health in Postmenopausal Women."

38. Chambers and Chaddha, "Effects of Whole Body Vibration Using the Vibrant Health Power 1000."

39. Chambers and Chaddha, "Effects of Whole Body Vibration Using the Vibrant Health Power 1000."

40. David Rossiaky, "Bone Density Scores for Osteoporosis," Healthline, February 21, 2023, https://www.healthline.com/health/t-score-vs-z-score-osteoporosis.

41. Kolata, "Low Buzz May Give Mice Better Bones and Less Fat."

42. C. T. Rubin et al., "Adipogenesis Is Inhibited by Brief, Daily Exposure to High-Frequency, Extremely Low-Magnitude Mechanical Signals," *Proceedings of the National Academy of Sciences* 104, no. 45 (2007): 17879–84, https://doi.org/10.1073/pnas.0708467104.

43. Clinton Rubin, Gang Xu, and Stefan Judex, "The Anabolic Activity of Hone Tissue, Suppressed by Disuse, Is Normalized by Brief Exposure to Extremely Low-Magnitude Mechanical Stimuli," *The FASEB Journal* 15 (October 2001), https://faseb.onlinelibrary.wiley.com/doi/epdf/10.1096/fj.01-0166com.

44. Y. X. Qin, C. T. Rubin, and K. J. McLeod, "Nonlinear Dependence of Loading Intensity and Cycle Number in the Maintenance of Bone Mass and Morphology," *Journal of Orthopaedic Research* 16, no. 4 (1998): 482-489, https://doi.org/10.1002/jor.1100160414.

45. Clinton Rubin et al., "Low Mechanical Signals Strengthen Long Bones." *Nature* 412 (2001): 603–604. https://doi.org/10.1038/35088122.

46. Ward et al., "Low Magnitude Mechanical Loading Is Osteogenic.".

47. T. P. Lam et al., "Effect of Whole Body Vibration (WBV) Therapy on Bone Density and Bone Quality in Osteopenic Girls with Adolescent Idiopathic Scoliosis: A Randomized, Controlled Trial," *Osteoporos International* 24 no. 5 (2013): 1623–1636, https://doi.org/10.1007/s00198-012-2144-1.

48. M. L. Bianchi et al., "Effects of Low-Magnitude High-Frequency Vibration on Bone Density, Bone Resorption and Muscular Strength in Ambulant Children Affected by Duchenne Muscular Dystrophy," *Journal of Bone and Mineral Research* 28, no. 5 (2013), https://www.cochranelibrary.com/central/doi/10.1002/central/CN-01064425/full.

49. Regina Dantas Jales de Oliveira et al., "Effectiveness of Whole-Body Vibration on Bone Mineral Density in Postmenopausal Women: A Systematic Review and Meta-Analysis of Randomized Controlled Trials," *Osteoporosis International* 34 (2023): 29–52, https://doi.org/10.1007/s00198-022-06556-y.

50. Clinton Rubin et al., "Prevention of Postmenopausal Bone Loss by a Low-Magnitude, High-Frequency Mechanical Stimuli: A Clinical Trial Assessing Compliance, Efficacy, and Safety," *Journal of Bone Mineral Research* 19, no. 3 (2009): 343–51, https://doi.org/10.1359/JBMR.0301251.

51. Bihiyga Salhi et al., "Effects of Whole Body Vibration in Patients with COPD," *COPD: Journal of Chronic Obstructive Pulmonary Disease* 12, no. 5 (2015): 525–32, https://doi.org/10.3109/15412555.2015.1008693.

52. Vincente Gilsanz et al., "Low-Level, High-Frequency Mechanical Signals Enhance Musculoskeletal Development of Young Women with Low BMD," *Journal of Bone Mineral Research* 21, no. 9 (2009): 1464–74. https://doi.

org/10.1359/jbmr.060612. PMID: 16939405.

53. Lara Pizzorno et al., *Your Bones: How You Can Prevent Osteoporosis & Have Strong Bones for Life Naturally* (Mount Jackson, VA: Praktikos Books, 2011), 6.

54. Pizzorno, *Your Bones: How You Can Prevent Osteoporosis, 17–23.*

55. Pizzorno, Your Bones: *How You Can Prevent Osteoporosis*, 31–40.

56. Belinda Beck, "The Effect of Low-Intensity Whole-Body Vibration with or without High-Intensity Resistance and Impact Training on Risk Factors for Proximal Femur Fragility Fracture in Postmenopausal Women with Low Bone Mass: Study Protocol for the VIBMOR Randomized Controlled Trial," *Trials* 23, no. 1 (2022): 15, https://doi.org/10.1186/s13063-021-05911-4.

57. Gabriel M. Pagnotti et al., "Combating Osteoporosis and Obesity with Exercise: Leveraging Cell Mechanosensitivity," *Nature Reviews Endocrinology* 15 (2019): 339–355, https://doi.org/10.1038/s41574-019-0170-1.

58. Pizzorno, *Your Bones: How You Can Prevent Osteoporosis*, 134.

59. Pizzorno, *Your Bones: How You Can Prevent Osteoporosis*, 67.

60. Kagaku Azuma et al., "Chronic Psychological Stress as a Risk Factor of Osteoporosis," *Journal of UOEH* 37, no. 4 (2015): 245–53. https://doi.org/102.7888/juoeh.37.245.

61. Pizzorno, *Your Bones: How You Can Prevent Osteoporosis*, 165.

62. Martie Whittekin, *Natural Alternatives to Nexium, Maalox, Tagamet, Prilosec & Other Acid Blockers: What to Use to Relieve Acid Reflux, Heartburn, and Gastric Ailments*, 2nd edition (Garden City Park, NY: Square One Publishers, 2009), 4–6.

63. National Institutes of Health, "Vitamin D Fact Sheet for Consumers," accessed September 20, 2023, https://ods.od.nih.gov/pdf/factsheets/VitaminD-Consumer.pdf.

Chapter 4

64. Gretchen Reynolds, "Jogging Your Brain," The *New York Times Magazine*, April 18, 2012, https://www.nytimes.com/2012/04/22/magazine/how-exercise-could-lead-to-a-better-brain.html.

65. Makoto Ariizumi and Akira Okada, "Effect of Whole Body Vibration on the Rat Brain Content of Serotonin and Plasma Corticosterone," *European Journal of Applied Physiology and Occupational Physiology* 52, no. 1 (1983): 15–19, https://doi.org/10.1007/bf00429019.

66. Yingjun Nie et al., "Association between Physical Exercise and Mental Health during the COVID-19 Outbreak in China: A Nationwide Cross-Sectional Study," *Psychiatry*. 12 (August 16, 2021), https://doi.org/10.3389/fpsyt.2021.722448.

67. Bosco et al., "Hormonal Responses to Whole-Body Vibration in Men."

68. Ariizumi and Okada, "Effect of Whole Body Vibration on the Rat Brain Content of Serotonin and Plasma Corticosterone."

69. Geetangli Chawla et al., "Effect of Whole-Body Vibration on Depression, Anxiety, Stress, and Quality of Life in College Students: A Randomized Controlled Trial," *Oman Medical Journal* 37, no. 4 (2022): e408, https://doi.org/10.5001/omj.2022.72.

70. Heidrun Lioba Wunram et al., "Whole Body Vibration Added to Treatment As Usual Is Effective in Adolescents with Depression: A Partly Randomized, Three-Armed Clinical Trial in Inpatients," *European Child & Adolescent Psychiatry* 27 (2018): 645–62, https://doi.org/10.1007/s00787-017-1071-2.

71. Anas R. Alashram, Elvira Padua, and Giuseppe Annino, "Effects of Whole-Body Vibration on Motor Impairments in Patients with Neurological Disorders: A Systematic Review," *American Journal of Physical Medicine & Rehabilitation* 98, no. 12 (2019): 1084–98, https://doi.org/10.1097/PHM.0000000000001252. PMID: 31246611.

72. Christina Brogårdh, Ulla-Brit Flansbjer, and Jan Lexell, "No Specific Effect of Whole-Body Vibration Training in Chronic Stroke: A Double-Blind Randomized Controlled Study," *Archives of Physical Medicine and Rehabilitation* 93, no. 2 (2012):253–58, https://doi.org/ 10.1016/j.apmr.2011.09.005.

73. M. Y. C. Pang, R. W. K. Lau, and S. P. Yip, "The Effects of Whole-Body Vibration Therapy on Bone Turnover, Muscle Strength, Motor Function, and Spasticity in Chronic Stroke: A Randomized Controlled Trial," *European Journal of Physical Rehabilitation Medicine* 49, no. 4 (2013): 439–50, https://pubmed.ncbi.nlm.nih.gov/23486302/.

74. Christoph Hilgers et al., "Effects of Whole-Body Vibration Training on Physical Function in Patients with Multiple Sclerosis," *NeuroRehabilitation* 32, no. 3 (2013): 655–63. https://doi.org/10.3233/NRE-130888.

75. Hsin-Yi Kathy Cheng et al., "Effects of an Eight-Week Whole Body Vibration on Lower Extremity Muscle Tone and Function in Children with Cerebral Palsy," *Research in Developmental Disabilities* 38 (2015): 256–61, https://doi.org/10.1016/j.ridd.2014.12.017.

76. Oliver Kaut et al., "Postural Stability in Parkinson's Disease Patients Is Improved after Stochastic Resonance Therapy," *Parkinson's Disease* 2016 (2016), https://doi.org/10.1155/2016/7948721.

77. Stephan Turbanski et al., "Effects of Random Whole-Body Vibration on Postural Control in Parkinson's Disease," *Research in Sports Medicine* 13, no. 3 (2005): 243–56, https://doi.org/10.1080/15438620500222588.

78. Brogårdh, Flansbjer, and Lexell, "No Specific Effect of Whole-Body Vibration Training in Chronic Stroke."

79. Ilse J. W. van Nes et al. "Long-Term Effects of 6-Week Whole-Body Vibration on Balance Recovery and Activities of Daily Living in the Postacute Phase of Stroke: A Randomized, Controlled Trial," *Stroke* 37, no. 9 (2006): 2331–35, https://doi.org/10.1161/01.STR.0000236494.62957.f3.

80. Ekaterina Tankisheva et al., "Effects of Intensive Whole-Body Vibration Training on Muscle Strength and Balance in Adults with Chronic Stroke: A

Randomized Controlled Pilot Study," *Archives of Physical Medicine Rehabilitation* 95, no. 3 (2013): 439–46, https://doi.org/10.1016/j.apmr.2013.09.009.

81. Othmar Schuhfried et al., "Effects of Whole-Body Vibration in Patients with Multiple Sclerosis: A Pilot Study," *Clinical Rehabilitation* 19, no. 8 (2005): 834–42, https://doi.org/10.1191/0269215505cr919oa.

82. Anselm B. M. Fuermaier et al., "Good Vibrations – Effects of Whole Body Vibration on Attention in Healthy Individuals and Individuals with ADHD," PLoS One 9, no. 2 (2014): e90747, https://doi.org/10.1371/journal.pone.0090747.

83. Ki-Hong Kim and Hyang-Beum Lee, "The Effects of Whole Body Vibration Exercise Intervention on Electroencephalogram Activation and Cognitive Function in Women with Senile Dementia," Journal of Exercise Rehabilitation 14, no. 4 (2018): 586–91, https://doi.org/10.12965/jer.1836230.115.

84. Lucrezia Moggio et al., "Vibration Therapy Role in Neurological Diseases Rehabilitation: An Umbrella Review of Systematic Reviews," *Disability and Rehabilitation* 44, no. 20 (2022): 5741–49, https://doi.org/10.1080/0963828 8.2021.1946175.

85. Cheng et al., "Effects of an Eight-Week Whole Body Vibration on Lower Extremity."

86. Lotta Ahlborg, Christina Andersson, and Per Julin, "Whole-Body Vibration Training Compared with Resistance Training: Effect on Spasticity, Muscle Strength and Motor Performance in Adults with Cerebral Palsy," *Journal of Rehabilitation Medicine* 38, no. 5 (2006): 302–8, https://doi.org/10.1080/16501970600680262.

87. Hilgers et al., "Effects of Whole-Body Vibration Training on Physical Function in Patients with Multiple Sclerosis."

88. I. M. Alguacil Diego et al., "Efectos de la Vibroterapia Sobre el Control Postural, la Funcionalidad y la Fatiga en Pacientes con Esclerosis Múltiple: Ensayo Clínico Aleatorizado [Effects of Vibrotherapy on Postural Control, Functionality and Fatigue in Multiple Sclerosis Patients: A Randomised Clinical Trial]," *Neurología* 27, no. 3 (2012): 143–53, Spanish, https://doi.org/10.1016/j.nrl.2011.04.019.

89. Georg Ebersbach et al., "Whole Body Vibration versus Conventional Physiotherapy to Improve Balance and Gait in Parkinson's Disease," *Archives of Physical Medicine and Rehabilitation* 89, no. 3 (March 2008): 399–403, https://doi.org/10.1016/j.apmr.2007.09.031.

90. Patricia Hannon. "Vibrating Glove Shows Promise for Calming Parkinson's Symptoms," SCOPE: Stanford Medicine. November 24, 2021.

91. Peter A. Tass, "Vibrotactile Coordinated Reset Stimulation for the Treatment of Parkinson's Disease," *Neural Regeneration Research* 17, no. 7 (July 2022): 1495–97, https://doi.org/10.4103/1673-5374.329001.

92. Anthony J. Martorell et al., "Multi-sensory Gamma Stimulation Ameliorates Alzheimer's-Associated Pathology and Improves Cognition," Cell 177,

no. 2 (March 14, 2019): 256–71, e22..

93. Anne Trafton, "Synchronized Brain Waves Enable Rapid Learning: MIT Study Finds Neurons That Hum Together Encode New Information," MIT News, June 12, 2014.

94. Fuermaier et al., "Good Vibrations – Effects of Whole Body Vibration on Attention."

95. Francisca Monteiro et al., "Multi-Mechanical Waves against Alzheimer's Disease Pathology: A Systematic Review," Translational Neurodegeneration 10, no. 1 (2021): 36, https://doi.org/10.1186/s40035-021-00256-z.

96. Trafton, "Synchronized Brain Waves Enable Rapid Learning."

97. Trafton, "Synchronized Brain Waves Enable Rapid Learning."

98. Trafton, "Synchronized Brain Waves Enable Rapid Learning."

99. Joe Dispenza, Becoming Supernatural: How Common People Are Doing the Uncommon (Carlsbad, CA: Hay House, 2017), 67.

100. Dispenza, Becoming Supernatural, 65–7.

101. Keith DeOrio, Vibranetics: The Complete Whole Body Vibration Fitness Solution (Santa Monica, CA: self-published, 2008), 31.

102. Bosco et al., "Hormonal Responses to Whole-Body Vibration in Men."

Chapter 5

103. Norman Shealy and Dawson Church, Soul Medicine: Awakening Your Inner Blueprint for Abundant Health and Energy (Santa Rosa, CA: Elite Books, 2006), 208–12.

104. Shealy and Church, Soul Medicine, 16.

105. Shealy and Church, Soul Medicine, 16.

106. Richard Gerber, Vibrational Medicine: The #1 Handbook of Subtle-Energy Therapies, 3rd edition (Rochester, NY: Bear and Co., 2001), 53–6.

107. American Association of Acupuncture and Bio-Energetic Medicine, "Basic Explanation of the Electrodermal Screening Test and the Concepts of Bio-Energetic Medicine."

108. Shealy and Church, Soul Medicine, 206.

109. Shealy and Church, Soul Medicine, 212.

110. Shealy and Church, Soul Medicine, 213.

111. Shealy and Church, Soul Medicine, 212.

112. Lauren Terhorst et al., "Complementary and Alternative Medicine in the Treatment of Pain in Fibromyalgia: A Systematic Review of Randomized Controlled Trials," Journal of Manipulative and Psychological Therapeutics 34, no. 7 (September 2011): 483–96, https://doi.org/10.1016/j.jmpt.2011.05.006.

113. Gerber, Vibrational Medicine,

114. Nadya M. Dhanani, Thomas J. Caruso, and Adam J. Carinci, "Complementary and Alternative Medicine for Pain: An Evidence-Based Review," Current Pain and Headache Reports 15, no.1 2011): 39–46, https://doi.org/10.1007/s11916-010-0158-y.

115. Joseph M. Day and Arthur J. Nitz, "The Effect of Muscle Energy Techniques on Disability and Pain Scores in Individuals with Low Back Pain," *Journal of Sport Rehabilitation* 21, no. 2 (May 2012): 194–8, https://doi.org/10.1123/jsr.21.2.194.

116. Bill Reddy, "Insights with Norm Shealy," *Acupuncture Today* 13, no. 6 (June 2012), https://www.acupuncturetoday.com/mpacms/at/article.php?id=32580.

117. Jack C. Yu et al., "Pain and Management of Pain: A Clinical Review for Craniofacial Surgeons," *Sage Journals* 2, no. 2 (May 2021), https://doi.org/10.1177%2F27325016211009271.

Chapter 6

118. "Depression and Pain. Hurting Bodies and Suffering Minds Often Require the Same Treatment," *Harvard Mental Health Letter* 3 (September 21, 2004): 4–5, PMID: 15381481.

119. Yi-Li Zheng et al., "Effect of 12-Week Whole-Body Vibration Exercise on Lumbopelvic Proprioception and Pain Control in Young Adults with Non-specific Low Back Pain," *Medical Science Monitor* 25 (2019): 443–52, https://doi.org/10.12659/MSM.912047.

120. T. S. Kaeding et al., "Whole-Body Vibration Training as a Workplace-Based Sports Activity for Employees with Chronic Low-Back Pain," *Scandinavian Journal of Medicine & Science in Sports* 27, no. 12 (2017): 2027–39, https://doi.org/10.1111/sms.12852.

121. Jörn Rittweger et al., "Treatment of Chronic Lower Back Pain with Lumbar Extension and Whole-Body Vibration Exercise: A Randomized Controlled Trial," *Spine* 27, no. 17 (September 2002): 1829–34, https://doi.org/10.1097/00007632-200209010-00003.

122. Borja del Pozo-Cruz et al., "Effects of Whole Body Vibration Therapy on Main Outcome Measures for Chronic Non-Specific Low Back Pain: A Single-Blind Randomized Controlled Trial," *Journal of Rehabilitation Medicine* 43, no. 8 (2011): 689–94, https://doi.org/10.2340/16501977-0830.

123. Achim Elfering et al., "Acute Effects of Stochastic Resonance Whole Body Vibration," *World Journal of Orthopedics* 4, no. 4 (October 18, 2013): 291–98, https://doi.org/10.5312/wjo.v4.i4.291.

124. Julia Bidonde et al., "Whole Body Vibration Exercise Training for Fibromyalgia," *Cochrane Database of Systematic Reviews* (September 26, 2017), https://doi.org/10.1002/14651858.CD011755.pub2.

125. Bidonde et al., "Whole Body Vibration Exercise Training for Fibromyalgia."

126. Nathan J. Kessler, Michael M. Lockard, and Jacob Fischer, "Whole Body Vibration Improves Symptoms of Diabetic Peripheral Neuropathy," *Prevention and Rehabilitation* 24, No. 2 (2020): 1–3, https://doi.org/10.1016/j.jbmt.2020.01.004.

127. Albina Jamal et al., "Whole Body Vibration Showed Beneficial Effect on Pain, Balance Measures and Quality of Life in Painful Diabetic Peripheral Neuropathy: A Randomized Controlled Trial," *Journal of Diabetes & Metabolic Disorders* 19 (2020): 61–9, https://doi.org/10.1007/s40200-019-00476-1.

128. Jamal et al., "Whole Body Vibration Showed Beneficial Effect on Pain."

129. Chen Guang Qiu et al., "Effects of Whole-Body Vibration Therapy on Knee Osteoarthritis: A Systematic Review and Meta-Analysis of Randomized Controlled Trials. Journal of Rehabilitation Medicine 54, (2022), https://www.doi.org/10.2340/jrm.v54.2032.

130. Hamid Reza Bokaeian et al., "The Effect of Adding Whole Body Vibration Training to Strengthening Training in the Treatment of Knee Osteoarthritis: A Randomized Clinical Trial," *Journal of Bodywork and Movement Therapies* 20, no. 2 (April 2016): 334–40, https://doi.org/10.1016/j.jbmt.2015.08.005.

131. Young Geun Park et al., "Therapeutic Effect of Whole Body Vibration on Chronic Knee Osteoarthritis," *Annals of Rehabilitation Medicine* 37, no. 4 (2013): 505–15, https://doi.org/10.5535/arm.2013.37.4.505.

132. Adriano P. Simão et al., "Functional Performance and Inflammatory Cytokines after Squat Exercises and Whole-Body Vibration in Elderly Individuals with Knee Osteoarthritis," *Archives of Physical Medicine and Rehabilitation* 93, no. 10 (2012): 1692–1700, https://doi.org/10.1016/j.apmr.2012.04.017.

133. Taishi Tsuji et al., "Effects of Whole-Body Vibration Exercise on Muscular Strength and Power, Functional Mobility and Self-Reported Knee Function in Middle-Aged and Older Japanese Women with Knee Pain," *The Knee* 21, no. 6 (December 2014): 1088–95, https://doi.org/10.1016/j.knee.2014.07.015.

134. T. Trans et al., "Effect of Whole Body Vibration Exercise on Muscle Strength and Proprioception in Females with Knee Osteoarthritis," *The Knee* 16, no. 4 (August 2009): 256–61, https://doi.org/10.1016/j.knee.2008.11.014.

135. Nubia Carelli Pereira Avelar et al., "The Effect of Adding Whole-Body Vibration to Squat Training on the Functional Performance and Self-Report of Disease Status in Elderly Patients with Knee Osteoarthritis: A Randomized, Controlled Clinical Study," *Journal of Alternative and Complementary Medicine* 17, no. 12 (2011): 1149–55, https://doi.org/10.1089/acm.2010.0782.

136. Hamayun Zafar et al., "Therapeutic Effects of Whole-Body Vibration Training in Knee Osteoarthritis: A Systematic Review and Meta-Analysis," *Archives of Physical Medicine and Rehabilitation* 96, no. 8 (2015): 1525–32, https://doi.org/10.1016/j.apmr.2015.03.010.

137. Zafar et al., "Therapeutic Effects of Whole-Body Vibration Training in Knee Osteoarthritis."

138. Chambers and Chaddha, "Effects of Whole Body Vibration Using the Vibrant Health Power 1000."

Chapter 7

139. Jawed et al., "Whole-Body Vibration Training Increases Stem/Progenitor Cell Circulation."

140. Bosco et al., "Hormonal Responses to Whole-Body Vibration in Men."

141. Phuc Van Pham, "Stem Cell Drugs: The Next Generation of Pharmaceutical Products." *Biomedical Research and Therapy* 3, no. 10 (2016), https://doi.org/10.15419/bmrat.v3i10.128.

142. Jawed et al., "Whole-Body Vibration Training Increases Stem/Progenitor Cell Circulation."

143. Bosco et al., "Hormonal Responses to Whole-Body Vibration in Men."

144. S. Murphy et al., "Sex Hormones and Bone Mineral Density in Elderly Men," *Bone and Mineral* 20, no. 2 (1993): 133–40, https://doi.org/ 10.1016/ s0169-6009(08)80022-0.

145. P. J. Kelly et al., "Dietary Calcium, Sex Hormones, and Bone Mineral Density in Men," *British Medical Journal* 300, no. 6736 (May 26, 1990): 1361–64, https://doi.org/10.1136/bmj.300.6736.1361.

146. Gail A. Greendale, Sharon Edelstein, and Elizabeth Barrett-Connor, "Endogenous Sex Steroids and Bone Mineral Density in Older Women and Men: The Rancho Bernardo Study," *Journal of Bone and Mineral Research* 12, no. 11 (2009: 1833–43, https://doi.org/10.1359/jbmr.1997.12.11.1833.

147. Marialuisa Giunta et al., "Growth Hormone-Releasing Effects of Whole Body Vibration Alone or Combined with Squatting plus External Load in Severely Obese Female Subjects," *Obesity Facts* 5, no. 4 (2012): 567–74, https://doi.org/10.1159/000342066.

148. A. Sartorio et al., "Growth Hormone and Lactate Responses Induced by Maximal Isometric Voluntary Contractions and Whole-Body Vibrations in Healthy Subjects," *Journal of Endocrinological Investigation* 34, no. 3, (2011): 216–21, https://doi.org/10.1007/BF03347069.

149. Thue Kvorning et al., "Effects of Vibration and Resistance Training on Neuromuscular and Hormonal Measures," *European Journal of Applied Physiology* 96, no. 5 (2006): 615–25, https://doi.org/10.1007/s00421-006-0139-3.

150. Bosco et al., "Hormonal Responses to Whole-Body Vibration in Men."

151. Murphy et al., "Sex Hormones and Bone Mineral Density in Elderly Men."

152. Giunta et al., "Growth Hormone-Releasing Effects of Whole Body Vibration."

153. Sartorio et al., "Growth Hormone and Lactate Responses."

154. Kvorning et al., "Effects of Vibration and Resistance Training."

155. Susan Rako, MD, *The Hormone of Desire: The Truth about Testosterone, Sexuality, and Menopause* (New York: Three Rivers Press, 1996), 25.

156. John P. Cunha, "Androgel," RxList, last updated November 17, 2022, http://www.rxlist.com/androgel-side-effects-drug-center.htm.

157. Alfio Albasini, Martin Krause, and Ingo Rembitzki, *Using Whole Body*

Vibration in Physical Therapy and Sport: Clinical Practice and Treatment Exercises (Edinburgh, Scotland; Churchill Livingstone, 2010).

158. Bidonde et al., "Whole Body Vibration Exercise Training for Fibromyalgia."

159. Prioreschi, "In Patients with Established RA, Positive Effects."

160. Prioreschi, "In Patients with Established RA, Positive Effects."

161. Chambers and Chaddha, "Effects of Whole Body Vibration Using the Vibrant Health Power 1000."

Chapter 8

162. R. Tossige-Gomes et al., "Whole-Body Vibration Decreases the Proliferative Response of TCD4+ Cells in Elderly Individuals with Knee Osteoarthritis," *Brazilian Journal of Medical and Biological Research* 45, no. 12 (December 2012): 1262–68, https://doi.org/10.1590/S0100-879X2012007500139.

163. Yu et al., "Whole Body Vibration-Induced Omental Macrophage Polarization."

164. "Chemical Body Burden: Bill Moyers' Test Results," PBS, accessed September 15, 2023, http://www.pbs.org/tradesecrets/problem/bodyburden.html.

165. Sherry A. Rogers, M.D., *Detoxify or Die* (Sarasota, FL: Sand Key Co., 2002),

Francisca Monteiro et al., "Multi-Mechanical Waves against Alzheimer's Disease Pathology: A Systematic Review," Translational Neurodegeneration 10, no. 1 (2021): 36, https://doi.org/10.1186/s40035-021-00256-z.

About the Author

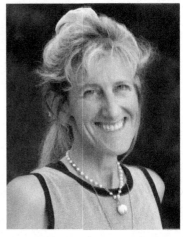

Becky Chambers is a natural health practitioner, teacher, author, and president and owner of Vibrant Health. She specializes in the breakthrough body, mind, and energy therapy of whole body vibration and the energy-medicine system of homeopathy. Ms. Chambers is a world expert in whole body vibration with twenty-five years of experience using and promoting it worldwide as an exercise and therapeutic system. This book is the second edition of her first book on the subject (first released in 2013), and it has been a best-seller ever since. Ms. Chambers has a bachelor of science degree in biology from the University of Massachusetts, a master's in education from Lesley College, and a graduate degree in natural health, specializing in homeopathy from Clayton College of Natural Health.

She has spent the last forty years discovering powerful new therapies, focusing particularly on whole body vibration and homeopathy, that have led to a transformation of her life on every level. She has published five other books, *Whole Body Vibration for Calming Inflammation, Whole Body Vibration for Mental Health, Whole Body Vibration for Seniors, Homeopathy Plus Whole Body Vibration, and Beyond the Great Abyss: A True Story of Transformation through Natural Health Breakthroughs* (a memoir not currently in print). Becky Chambers is also available for consultations. To work with her, please contact her through her website at:

www.BCVibrantHealth.com

Printed in Great Britain
by Amazon

38347530R00126